Table of Contents

TABLE OF CONTENTS   **three**

INTRODUCTION   **one**

1. INITIAL ASSESSMENT OF INFORMATION NEEDS   **three**

Why install a nursing management system?   three

Problems   six

A way forward   nine

Which functions?   seventeen

2. CARE PLANNING   **nineteen**

The potential benefits of computerisation   nineteen

Problems associated with computer assisted care planning   twenty

A way forward   twenty-three

Better use of care planning systems   twenty-five

3. WORKLOAD ASSESSMENT   **twenty-seven**

The potential benefits   twenty-seven

Problems   twenty-eight

Workload assessment – a way forward   forty

Reviewing existing workload assessment systems   forty-four

4. ROSTERING   **forty-seven**

The potential benefits of computerisation   forty-seven

Problems .... forty-eight

A way forward .... fifty-one

5. IMPLEMENTATION & EVALUATION   **fifty-five**

Problems .... fifty-five

Successful implementation .... fifty-seven

In conclusion .... sixty-two

SUMMARY OF RECOMMENDATIONS: **sixty-three**

For hospitals that have not yet finalised their choice of nursing system:
    sixty-three

For hospitals which already have a nursing management system   sixty-six

REFERENCES   **sixty-nine**

APPENDIX 1   **seventy-one**

Acknowledgements .... seventy-one

APPENDIX 2   **seventy-five**

Glossary .... seventy-five

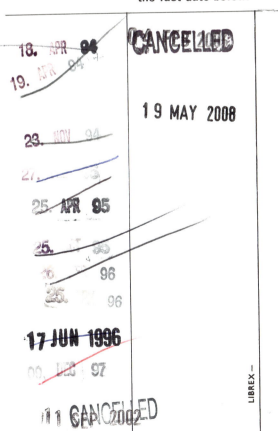
Caring Systems:
Effective Implementation of Ward Nursing Management Systems

A Handbook for Managers
of Nursing and Project
Managers

LONDON: HMSO

0118860909

© Crown copyright 1992

Applications for reproduction should be made to HMSO

First published December 1992

Printed in the UK for the Audit Commission by Press-on-Printers Ltd
ISBN 011 886 0909

London : HMSO

Audit Commission, National Health Service Handbook

Introduction

1. The purpose of this handbook is to help project nurses and others choose and implement a ward nursing management and information system (NMS) that will not just help nurses do their jobs more efficiently, but will also to enable them to care for patients better within available resources. It is called 'Caring Systems' because frequently nurses and their managers do not see how a NMS could help them with changes that they would like to make to improve the quality of care. It is the second handbook on nursing in acute general wards to be published by the Audit Commission in succession to its report 'The Virtue of Patients' (Ref. 1). That report recommends an agenda of action for senior hospital managers to improve the effectiveness and efficiency of nursing services in co-operation with ward staff. The first handbook, 'Making Time for Patients' (Ref. 2), goes on to show how ward sisters and their immediate managers can emulate existing good practice which has demonstrably improved the quality of patient care.

2. Like 'The Virtue of Patients', this handbook is based on discussions with nurses from 39 general medical, general surgical and acute care of the elderly wards and on analysis of the data and documents which they provided. These have been supplemented by study of literature and by visits to other acute hospitals using a wide range of different nursing systems in England and Wales, France and the USA. The systems themselves continue to evolve, but the principles underlying how they can best be used do not change significantly. This handbook does not however cover the use of systems in other settings such as theatres or the community. Nor do all of the observations made necessarily apply in longer-stay hospital settings where nursing workload and the care needs of patients may be more stable than in acute wards. The handbook is confined to 'nursing systems', because such professional divisions reflect the way in which development is currently funded and planned in most hospitals. However it fully subscribes to the ideal that 'information systems should be based on the individual patient and be used by all health care staff, irrespective of profession, in order to support the provision of high quality, collaborative, seamless care'.

Exhibit 1

THE STRUCTURE OF THIS HANDBOOK

1

Initial Assessment of information needs

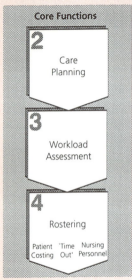

Core Functions

2

Care Planning

3

Workload Assessment

4

Rostering

Patient Costing | 'Time Out' | Nursing Personnel

5

Implementation & Evaluation

Source: Audit Commission

3. It is written with the benefit of hindsight! If, in places, it appears critical of current systems or the way in which they are used, the intention is not to decry the work of those nurses and managers who have led the way in this field, but to draw attention to potential pitfalls that have since emerged and ways in which others can avoid them. Recent audits have confirmed that many hospitals have yet to make a final choice of nursing system. They have also shown that in most others the concerns raised in this handbook remain valid. For these, such warnings may appear to come too late. However they should provoke thought about ways in which existing systems and procedures could be modified to make them more responsive to the needs of patients. They also emphasise the need to ensure that existing systems and their effects on patient care are evaluated periodically.

4. This handbook complements guidance on selecting and implementing nursing management systems issued during recent years by the Department of Health and by health service consultancies (Refs. 3 – 5) and current Procurement Guidelines for the NHS and Suppliers. The 'Step by Step' Guide to the Selection of a NMS published by Greenhalgh and Co for the King's Fund is particularly commended to those preparing the Statement of Need (or Operational Requirement) for a system. The descriptions contained in the same publisher's Guide to Current and Potential Systems will assist in the selection of potential suppliers. The workload and skill mix volumes of the 'Rainbow Pack' training material prepared by Regions to raise nurses' awareness of underlying resource management issues are also relevant (Ref. 6).

5. Section 1 of this handbook starts one step back from those publications by considering what factors need to be considered *before* starting to plan the acquisition of a ward nursing system (Exhibit 1). Sections two to four take a separate look at three core NMS functions:- care planning, workload assessment and rostering. In each case, the ideal is reviewed, then problems, which have arisen at study sites are discussed and finally good practice is recommended. Section five is about choosing the system that is right for your hospital, its successful implementation and the evaluation of whether objectives have been achieved. A summary of recommendations is given at the end of the handbook.

Caring systems

Initial Assessment of Information Needs

WHY INSTALL A NURSING MANAGEMENT SYSTEM?

6. Almost half of health authorities' salary expenditure is for nursing. General nursing on acute hospital wards alone costs some £1.2 billions per year. Efficient and effective use of this major resource is vital to good patient care and to public perceptions of the quality of the NHS. The Audit Commission report 'The Virtue of Patients' argues that it is essential to manage wards and hospital nursing services in a way which promotes a more patient centred approach and greater continuity of care. It recommends staged adoption of the principles underlying primary nursing. To achieve this effectively, it advocates a move towards flexible use of more stable ward staffing, devolved responsibility for management of budgets and professional development of staff, coupled with structured systems for quality assurance. Good information about patients' needs and the resources required to satisfy them, about the way nurses are currently utilised and about the quality of care provided is vital if such moves are to be successful.

7. The core elements of current computerised ward nursing management and information systems[1] are:

▼   Care Planning and Evaluation,

▼   Workload Assessment,

▼   Rostering (planning and evaluation) including:
    Nursing Personnel and Time-Out Analyses.

---

1   The distinction between nursing management and nursing information systems is more of intent than
     of function. The terms are used interchangeably in this handbook.

8. These are the functions principally covered in this handbook. Each can also be performed manually and the relative advantages of computerisation must be weighed carefully. Although these functions do not meet all nursing information needs, they can help to answer a wide range of questions. For instance, how many ward staff are needed to ensure that all patients receive a good standard of nursing care? Are available nursing resources being used as efficiently and effectively as possible? What is the best skill mix for each ward? How can nurses' time be released to enable qualified staff to spend more time with the patient? How much on average does it cost to nurse patients with specific clinical conditions or nursing problems?

Exhibit 2

WARD NURSING MANAGEMENT & INFORMATION SYSTEMS
The 3 core elements of nursing systems may link to other hospital systems,

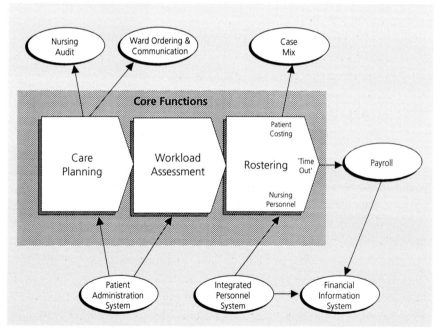

Source: Audit Commission

9. Computerised nursing management and information systems may also include Ward Ordering and Communication, allowing nurses for example to access the results of clinical tests or order drugs through ward based computer terminals. They may enable certain Patient Administration functions to be performed on the ward. Computers are increasingly used by qualified nurses and students for distance-learning, for nursing audit and research purposes. Some hospitals are developing multidisciplinary clinical systems. Systems are becoming available for monitoring a patient's progress against a profile of the care which he is likely to need and an anticipated recovery timetable. Nursing systems may also link with, for example, an Integrated Patient System, Payroll, a General Personnel System or a Case-Mix Management System (Exhibit 2). And, as nursing budgets are further devolved, it will be necessary for ward nurses to have on-line access to financial information systems.

10. Integrated hospital systems which cover a number of these areas are increasingly available, although still relatively costly. But many of the computerised nursing management systems currently in use perform only a subset of even the core functions. Of the ten hospitals studied in detail, four had introduced computer assisted care planning on at least some wards, four computerised workload assessment and three computerised rostering. Daily workload was calculated manually on some wards at two of the other hospitals. Just one of the additional hospitals visited was making full use of an integrated system. However, most of these routinely assessed workload by some means and one had automated rostering.

11. Great impetus was given to the pace of development and installation of computerised nursing systems by the Department of Health's timetable for introduction of Resource Management. Hospitals were urged to place an order for a nursing system by the end of their second year of funding and implement the system by the end of the third year. In some areas, this recommendation was interpreted prescriptively. Nevertheless, faced with a plethora of competing interests, changing methodologies and suppliers, many hospitals are still hesitating (Exhibit 3). For many of the pioneers, the promised benefits of installing a nursing management system are proving elusive. Others have felt in retrospect that they did not give sufficient time to choosing a solution that will be robust in the face of the changes occurring in nursing and in the NHS at present.

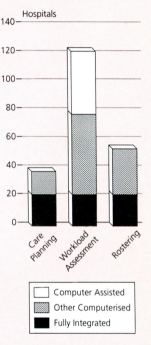

Exhibit 3

USE OF NURSING MANAGEMENT SYSTEMS IN MAJOR ACUTE GENERAL HOSPITALS
Many hospitals are still hesitating

Legend:
- Computer Assisted
- Other Computerised
- Fully Integrated

Source: *Audit Commission Estimates based on information from suppliers and audit returns*

PROBLEMS

(i) MEETING YESTERDAY'S NEEDS

12.   The first generation of nursing management systems often appears to have been introduced piecemeal rather than as part of a holistic plan for meeting the information needs of the service and helping it develop.   Information is often geared to the perceived needs of old-style line management, even where new, slimmer management structures have been introduced, rather than to the needs of ward nurses acting as responsible professionals. This was also noted by Keen and Malby (Ref. 7): 'At the (resource management) pilot sites, systems were imposed rather than being agreed through discussion, and reports thus held by senior nurse managers rather than being fed up from wards. The opportunity for nurses to establish proper professional management and clinical reporting arrangements was thus lost'.

13. There has been insufficient assessment of the changing needs of the service and the significance of emerging trends in the way nursing care is provided has not always been recognised when planning new systems. The 'named nurse' initiative heralded in the patients' charter, for instance, puts more emphasis on the need to retain continuity of care when rostering and allocating staff. To quote the 'Step by Step Guide' (Ref. 3): 'it is foolish for the nurses to describe their information requirements as they are currently, when there are major structural and organisational changes in the offing. The trouble is that frequently the service is in such a state of flux that staff really do not know what will be required of them in the future'. 'Some will find that' .. 'the impetus to install systems is somewhat in front of organisational change and the management of that change'.

(ii)   DIFFERING PERSPECTIVES AND INACCURATE ASSUMPTIONS

14. Two very distinct philosophical approaches to defining information needs have been observed. One views the prime purpose of nursing management systems as providing the information which ward nurses need about their patients if care is to be better managed, organised and assessed. The other concentrates on the information perceived to be needed for both day to day and longer term management and deployment of nursing staff.   Expectations of what would be achieved by

installing a NMS vary. Ward nurses, nurse managers and general management may have markedly different priorities and perspectives (Exhibit 4).

Exhibit 4

EXPECTATIONS OF A NURSING MANAGEMENT SYSTEM
Ward nurses, nurse managers and general management may have markedly different priorities and perspectives

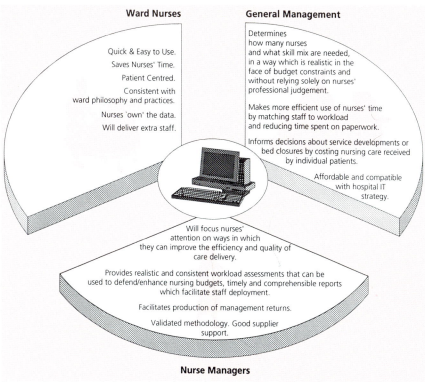

Ward Nurses

Quick & Easy to Use.
Saves Nurses' Time.
Patient Centred.
Consistent with ward philosophy and practices.
Nurses 'own' the data.
Will deliver extra staff.

General Management

Determines how many nurses and what skill mix are needed, in a way which is realistic in the face of budget constraints and without relying solely on nurses' professional judgement.

Makes more efficient use of nurses' time by matching staff to workload and reducing time spent on paperwork.

Informs decisions about service developments or bed closures by costing nursing care received by individual patients.

Affordable and compatible with hospital IT strategy.

Will focus nurses' attention on ways in which they can improve the efficiency and quality of care delivery.

Provides realistic and consistent workload assessments that can be used to defend/enhance nursing budgets, timely and comprehensible reports which facilitate staff deployment.

Facilitates production of management returns.

Validated methodology. Good supplier support.

Nurse Managers

Source: Audit Commission

15. Expectations are further confused because what *actually* happens on the wards now can be very different from what some senior nurses and managers *think* happens. Care and discharge plans for instance may be completed only perfunctorily. Many of the constraints and preferences that are taken into consideration when nurses construct 'off-duties' are implicit rather than stated. There can be considerable

variation in practice from ward to ward. Systems have sometimes been specified without a proper appreciation of the implications of these differences.

(iii) UNCLEAR OBJECTIVES

16. Few hospitals have specified objectives for their nursing management systems with sufficient clarity for impartial evaluation of their effectiveness to be possible. Where targets have been set, they have tended to relate to the technical functioning of the system and the processes of data entry. Broader objectives for the contribution that the system makes to quality of care and efficient management of ward resources are usually lacking.

17. At some hospitals, there has been an over-emphasis on listing all the types of data that nurses could possibly ever desire rather than on defining *what* additional information and new procedures are needed and *how* these would be used to improve resource management and quality of care. There has been insufficient prioritisation of functions, many of which, care audit facilities for example, have often proved to be too resource-intensive to use in practice.

(iv) 'LETTING THE TAIL WAG THE DOG'

18. A number of the hospitals studied had started from the presumption that a *computerised* nursing system was needed. Only then was consideration given to possible uses. The resulting systems constrain rather than facilitate changes that nurses subsequently wish to make to the organisation and quality of care. For example, some hospitals have:

▼ a computerised care planning system which restricts the extent to which plans can be individualised,

▼ a workload assessment system geared to moving pairs of hands around the hospital rather than to helping nurses plan their workload effectively,

▼ a rostering system which can not produce 'off-duties' that provide a satisfactory level and mix of staffing for each team of nurses within a ward.

Once implemented, it is harder to change a computerised system than to amend manual procedures.

(v) INCOMPLETE COSTINGS

19. The full costs of implementing and running a computerised system have seldom been evaluated. Whichever system is chosen, the cost of the nursing time needed to implement, support and operate it during its life-time is likely to be considerably greater than that spent on purchase and installation. If two minutes is spent per patient each day entering data into the computer, the total discounted cost to a 500 bed hospital just of the nurses' time could be £450,000 in the first five years.

20. It is not easy to compare the relative purchase costs of different systems or approaches. Some systems are supplied with an integral package of consultancy time, whereas for others this is charged separately. Specific software and support have at times been made available without charge by regions or on a development and show-case basis. Hardware costs will depend on what computers and cabling are already available in the hospital or are planned for other applications, and on what configuration of equipment is adopted.

(vi) UNREALISED PROMISES

21. Computerised products are constantly evolving. Many have only a very short track record by which purchasers can be guided. The number of additional facilities offered or promised, apparent ease of use and quality of report presentation can therefore assume inordinate importance when a system is chosen. Some hospitals have found that promises to add additional features or amend systems to meet local requirements have not been met within an acceptable timescale. There has also been disappointment in the quality of support and advice from some system suppliers.

A WAY FORWARD

(i) PUTTING INFORMATION SYSTEMS INTO CONTEXT

22. Systems should be planned in the context of patient care needs and the overall development of both the nursing service and the hospital (Exhibit 5). They must not be allowed to dictate or constrain ward organisation or clinical practice. The objective of an NMS review should not be seen simply to be computerisation of existing data flows. Professional initiatives to improve care need to be taken into consideration, as well as any forthcoming organisational reorganisation. Provision of better information is likely to be only one aspect of the changes required. Nurses

Exhibit 5

INITIAL ASSESSMENT
Information systems should be planned in the context of the overall development needs of the nursing service

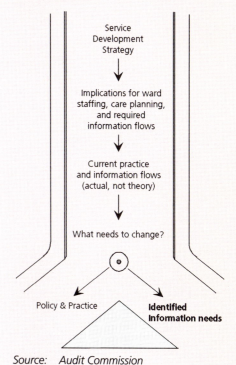

Service Development Strategy

Implications for ward staffing, care planning, and required information flows

Current practice and information flows (actual, not theory)

What needs to change?

Policy & Practice

Identified Information needs

Source: Audit Commission

THE STAGES OF IMPLEMENTING A NURSING MANAGEMENT SYSTEM - AN ANALOGY

It may be helpful to think of the stages of choosing and implementing a NMS as similar to those of the *nursing process:* (Exhibit 6). For the purpose of this analogy, the nursing service and its staff should be thought of as the collective *'patient'*. Nurses would not normally plan nursing interventions without first making a structured assessment of the patient's condition, prognosis and needs. Similarly it is inappropriate to plan a nursing management system in isolation from consideration of problems faced by wards and managers in improving care and making more efficient use of resources. The technical intervention of improving information flows by installing a NMS is likely to be only one of the ingredients needed to achieve a successful outcome. The project group will need to adopt the hospital's nursing strategy as their *model of care*. This should ensure that the assessment is drawn up in consultation with *'the patient'*, that it is comprehensive, holistic and recognises the distinct individual needs of different areas of the hospital and groups of staff, whether or not they be potential direct NMS users.

The project group can now go on to plan action to alleviate those aspects of the problem that can be addressed by better information. Wherever possible they should do this in consultation with *'the patient'* (ward staff and their managers) and with other professions within the hospital. If the plan is to be implemented effectively, staff will need a common understanding of the purpose and potential of any new system.

Exhibit 6

CHOOSING AND IMPLEMENTING A NURSING MANAGEMENT SYSTEM
The stages of choosing and implementing a nursing management system are analogous to those of the Nursing Process

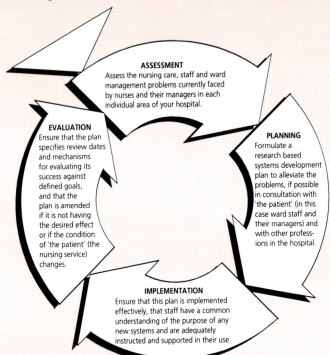

Source: Audit Commission

Education will be required in order to effect attitudinal change, if the ideals of resource management are to be attained. The plan should include specific measurable goals and review dates at which its success in meeting agreed objectives will be evaluated. If it does not have the desired effect or if the condition of 'the patient' changes, needs should be re-evaluated and the plan amended.

However it could be dangerous to pursue this analogy too far. Any systems development must be centred on the needs of the real patients rather than simply those of the staff or hospital management.

may find it helpful to consider whether there is a useful parallel between the stages of implementing a NMS and those of the *nursing process*. Both should comprise a cycle of assessment, planning, implementation and evaluation. This analogy is developed in Box A.

23. It is neither desirable nor practicable for a nursing systems project group to conduct a detailed review of the whole nursing strategy and operation of a hospital. But both the project group and the nursing staff who will be helping to define information requirements need to receive clear guidance from the Director of Nursing Services (DNS) as to how it is intended that the service will develop. Where there is no DNS at present, the 'Quality Nurse' and managers with responsibility for the quality of nursing care will perform this role. The local audits currently being carried out for the Audit Commission in many hospitals should help to crystalise these service development priorities. Their communication will be easier in those hospitals which have drawn up a coherent nursing development strategy and implementation plans co-ordinated with those for the hospital as a whole, as recommended in 'The Virtue of Patients'.

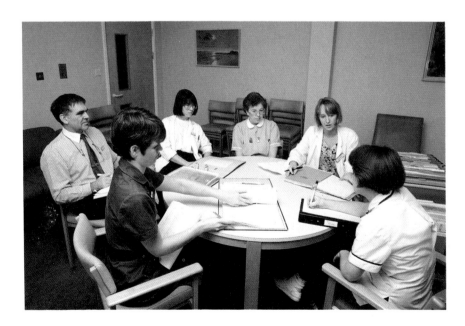

1 *Initial Assessment of Information Needs*

(ii) AN AGREED PHILOSOPHY AND APPRECIATION OF CURRENT PRACTICE

24. Hospitals need to be clear why they are introducing a Nursing Management System and who it is for. Agreement should be reached on the relative merits of differing information philosophies at the outset. Three American hospitals, selected for the quality of nursing care which they provide, were studied. At each, the firm emphasis is on information *for* nurses about patients and their needs – information which enables nurses to review their clinical practice – and on personnel and budgetary data for floor (ward) managers. Lesser priority is placed on generating information to regulate and monitor what nurses are doing. In the two French hospitals visited, clear guidelines had been agreed for the ways in which workload information would be used, primarily by nurses rather than by management.

25. With both this information philosophy and the nursing service strategy firmly in mind, the project group together with senior management should be in a position to reach broad conclusions about information needs. How will the information be used to improve resource usage and quality of care? The Director of Nursing Services should ensure that senior clinicians and the Unit Management Board concur with these conclusions and share a common commitment to the way forward.

26. Before starting to set out detailed system requirements, the project group needs to gain a detailed appreciation of current practice in such areas as care planning, rostering and staff management. The 'Step by Step Guide' includes a questionnaire that can be simplified where appropriate and used to help 'define the current situation'. The replies will provide the basis for consultation with ward staff as to which local practices must be accommodated by the proposed NMS and which can, or should, be modified. However nurses may find it difficult to describe what is distinctive about their wards and nursing practice unless they have sufficient knowledge about the way things are done elsewhere. Local audit reports may help by providing an independent source of information and comparison of ward practices.

(iii) A REALISTIC STATEMENT OF NEED AND CLEAR, PRIORITISED OBJECTIVES

27. Meticulous planning and adherence to sound project management procedures such as those described in the 'Step by Step Guide' (Ref. 3) is essential (Exhibit 7). It should start by considering how additional information would be used, when and by whom. What data need to be collected, in what detail and with what frequency? How can these best be processed into information and presented in the most easily assimilable way? How would this affect patients? Functions and additional system features should be prioritised in consultation with potential users of the system, but with due consideration of the resources that would be needed to make full use of

Exhibit 7

THE ROAD TO CHOOSING AN EFFECTIVE NURSING MANAGEMENT SYSTEM
Meticulous planning is essential

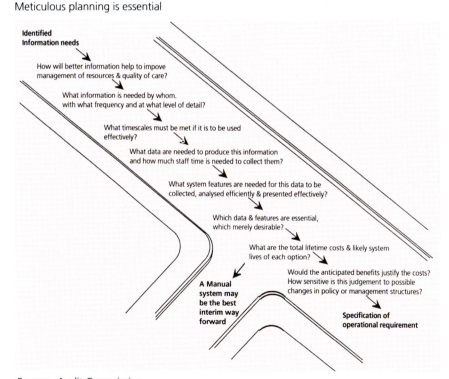

Identified Information needs

How will better information help to impove management of resources & quality of care?

What information is needed by whom. with what frequency and at what level of detail?

What timescales must be met if it is to be used effectively?

What data are needed to produce this information and how much staff time is needed to collect them?

What system features are needed for this data to be collected, analysed efficiently & presented effectively?

Which data & features are essential, which merely desirable?

What are the total lifetime costs & likely system lives of each option?

Would the anticipated benefits justify the costs? How sensitive is this judgement to possible changes in policy or management structures?

A Manual system may be the best interim way forward

Specification of operational requirement

Source: Audit Commission

them. A number of options should be developed and costed. If data will be provided and used by managers and staff from a number of different areas of the hospital, it can be helpful before choosing a system to 'model' its intended operation. A representative group should be brought together for a paper simulation of the operation of the preferred system and consequent actions. This can help to develop a shared appreciation of requirements and potential problems.

28. The scarcity of information available quantifying time savings and improvements in care achieved following the introduction of a NMS makes it even more important to agree clear objectives and specific related goals. Examples include:

▼ achieve full compliance with the hospital discharge policy;

▼ ensure that sensible review dates are set for all problems identified on care plans;

▼ increase the proportion of shifts on which a qualified nurse from each team is on duty;

▼ reduce the use of bank and agency nurses who have not previously worked on the ward;

▼ halve the time taken to produce payroll returns.

29. These objectives should complement such specific targets for system implementation and performance as the dates when the system will be introduced to each ward, response times, or the speed with which support is provided. The wider objectives should relate to issues which all groups of staff recognise as relevant and important. If this is not the case, major effort must be devoted finding out why this is so. Further professional development or inter-disciplinary seminars may be needed to broaden perspectives and change attitudes before implementation is worthwhile.

(vi) COMPUTERISED OR MANUAL – KEEP THE OPTIONS OPEN

30. Computerisation makes it feasible routinely to collect more detailed data and to analyse them in a more complex way for both management and research purposes. It may take time for the full benefits to be realised. Networked systems

enable nursing and patient data to be disseminated wider and faster, drawing on information from other linked systems as needed. They can also give management a better day to day overview. All the computerised information used by nurses should be accessible through the same ward terminals and information should be easily transferable between different systems. It may be intended that nursing data will eventually be fed into an integrated hospital information system. Emphasis on maintaining *open connection standards*, so that any supplier's systems and programs can be used, will help to ensure that this does not unduly constrain the choice of nursing system. Such plans may also affect the perceived balance of costs and benefits of computerising nursing information, but it is important to take a realistic view of potential future benefits. It must also be remembered that, no matter how sophisticated the processing, any information can only be as good as the quality of the data on which it is based.

31. However computerised nursing management systems should only be introduced if this is clearly the best way forward at the present time. The alternative of improving manual systems for use until nurses have a sufficiently clear, stable and well informed picture of ward information needs should also be examined.

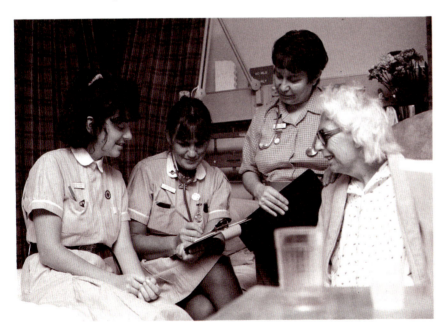

Manual systems are more flexible and capable of adaptation to individual patient needs. Depending on how they are implemented, they can also provoke more thought.

(v) ROBUST LIFE-CYCLE COSTING

32. Option costings should include the costs of setting up the system, training and educating staff, providing continuing support, collecting and processing the data, auditing the quality of information produced and evaluating the system. Costing the staff time required to operate the system during its lifetime is likely to suggest the choice of a system which is quick and easy to use. If the budget will not accommodate a suitable system, the best way forward may be to adopt a manual approach or to computerise only some of the desired functions. A temporary solution may be preferable to getting stuck with a monster that only partially meets its objectives. This should be presented to staff as a planned evolution. The broad philosophy underlying the interim solution should be similar to that of the system which it is envisaged that the hospital will eventually obtain so that the need for re-education is kept to a minimum.

33. Costs should be considered both in total and in comparison to those of present arrangements. The current rapid pace of system and other developments should be taken into account when estimating a realistic planned lifetime for each element of the system. How would the anticipated costs and benefits, both financial and quality improvements, be affected if different assumptions were made about system performance or the future of the service? What for instance would be the effect if responsibility for nursing were to be further devolved to clinical directorates or more authority delegated to ward sisters? What if interdisciplinary care planning, documentation and clinical audit became more of a reality? What if there were to be a marked change in nursing skill mix? What if shift patterns and rostering became more flexible? It may be safe to assume that, whatever happens, it will always be necessary to plan care, estimate workload, roster staff and cost the services provided to patients. But try if possible to make plans which are robust.

(vi) PROOF BEFORE PURCHASE OR IN-HOUSE DEVELOPMENT

34. In order to minimise problems with system suppliers when selecting or developing systems, full use should be made of any assistance available from health service

IT and management services professionals. Ensure that shortlisted suppliers understand your requirements and can meet them now, not at some indefinite future date. They must also have the capacity to provide adequate initial and continuing training and support.

35. If no suppliers can meet your statement of need and if time constraints permit, consider the option of an in-house development. Some hospitals have found this to be the best course. But it is necessary to proceed down this road with caution. If an in-house system is to be used cost-effectively by nurses, it must still be designed, programmed and documented to full commercial standards. With the current pace of technological change, further development of the system is likely to be required after implementation. It is essential to plan adequate resourcing for this. The possibilities of making use of such databases as libraries of care or intervention timings may be more restricted and so more input may be required from ward nurses to set up the system. Compatibility with data from other hospitals may be less. There will also be greater reliance on retaining the skills and experience of individuals to provide on-going system support.

WHICH FUNCTIONS?

36. Hospitals are coming to very different conclusions as to their requirements. Some Regions have, in the recent past, specified preferred systems to reduce cost and duplication of effort, concentrate expertise and improve the comparability of costings and workload information between hospitals. However it has proved difficult to ensure that systems are used in a comparable way. Also, the 1990 health service reforms have established such operational decisions to be the prerogative of local Trust or unit management. The regional or national role is best restricted to broad guidance. This ensures that systems are relevant to local needs and circumstances, so increasing commitment to use the information produced to improve practice.

37. There has been little evaluation of the extent to which any installed systems have produced the improvements which were expected. There is thus a lack of firm evidence for hospitals to draw upon when deciding which types of system would meet their needs most cost-effectively. The debate has been conducted in terms of what features appear to offer the most immediate benefits for staff and patients.

Which features would be most likely to secure and retain the commitment of all the nurses, doctors and managers who will need to act on the information produced by the system? Sections 2 to 4 of this handbook review problems that have arisen in making effective use of computer assisted care-planning, workload assessment and computerised rostering systems and recommend best practice. The considerations for each of these aspects are necessarily very different. Fundamentally, the key question for care planning and rostering is whether computerisation would improve the quality of plans or off-duties, and hence of patient care, whilst saving nurses' time. For workload assessment, it is first necessary to determine whether such information on a daily or shift basis is needed at all. Computerisation is a secondary consideration.

2

Care Planning

38. Planning the care needed by individual patients and its subsequent evaluation are essential components of the 'nursing process'. Their role in ensuring that patients are nursed efficiently and in improving the quality of care is developed in a companion handbook, 'Making Time for Patients'. The resulting care plans may also form part of the legal record of the care actually provided to each patient. This section evaluates the advantages and pitfalls of computerising these processes, or adopting alternative ways to make the more routine aspects of their production more efficient.

THE POTENTIAL BENEFITS OF COMPUTERISATION

39. Many senior nurses see care planning systems as the way into computerisation and nursing resource management which will produce the most obvious immediate benefits for nurses and patients alike. Their hope is that computerisation will save much of the time perceived to be spent by nurses in 'form filling', and that the completeness, consistency, timeliness and legibility of care plans will be improved. Nurses would be able to call up standard information at the touch of a button. More of their time could therefore be devoted to identifying the specific nursing, 'problems' presented by each individual patient, providing direct patient care, and assessing its effectiveness. The appeal of some care planning systems is broadened by the promise of 'management information' which, suppliers claim, will enable objective assessment of nursing workload based on 'timed' interventions. Further, this would be done in a way which neither requires time-consuming entry of further data nor is perceived by nurses as unduly constraining their professional judgements about patients' care needs.

40. In addition, care planning systems *potentially* provide a quality assurance tool. They could be a means of disseminating and monitoring compliance with research-

COMPUTER ASSISTED CARE PLANNING - A CASE STUDY

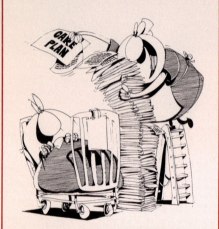

On one medical ward studied, the complete care plan of a patient staying for five or six weeks could amount to a pile of computer printout six inches thick. The way in which their system had been implemented forced full care plans for all patients on the ward, incorporating detailed standards for each intervention, to be reprinted daily, regardless of the amount of change. Any written individualisation was thus effectively lost the following day. A separate written continuation record of care was therefore necessary and all important information on the patient was held in this. The weight of the care plans precluded their use for handover between nurses. One side-room was completely filled with back care-plans. The impending storage crisis was to be resolved by using a scanner. Clinicians' views of the usefulness of nursing care plans were understandably scathing.

based nursing standards, a study aid for student nurses and an expert knowledge base for nurses faced with unusual nursing problems. A database for future nursing audit and research could be built up which would enable nursing interventions to be correlated with outcomes.

PROBLEMS ASSOCIATED WITH COMPUTER ASSISTED CARE PLANNING
(i) TIME AND EFFORT

41. Many hospitals have underestimated the considerable amount of nursing time required to set up and implement computer assisted care planning. Some packages provide only a shell into which the knowledge base, in the form of 'units of care' (nursing problems, activities and desired outcomes), must be entered locally before the system can be used. They rely heavily on groups of enthusiasts willing to devote time on top of their ward duties to setting up the system. Nurses thought that the guidance provided by some system suppliers was inappropriate. It was based on United States practice where nursing 'units of care' are heavily orientated towards medically driven interventions.

42. The potential benefits of computer assisted care planning in allowing the completeness and quality of care to be audited and for facilitating nursing audit have sometimes been a major factor in their selection. However at the hospitals studied, insufficient staff resources were available for details of the care *actually* delivered to be routinely fed back into the computer. No use therefore was made of any of the quality assurance and care audit modules.

(ii) CARE PLANS WHICH ARE DIFFICULT TO USE

43. Although the latest generation of systems is much more user-friendly than its predecessors, there is still considerable room for improvement. The format of computer output does not always encourage the use of care plans by nurses, other clinical staff and patients. Those studied were often too long [Box B], poorly laid out, and failed to highlight key problems. Where poor quality printers had been used, they were scarcely more legible than hand-written plans.

44. At some hospitals nurses are required to re-enter into the care planning system data already held on the patient administration system (PAS). This is clearly inefficient. However, problems can also arise where these systems are linked. At

one study site, the system had been specified in such a way that nurses were unable to complete a patient assessment or start to use the computer to plan care until patient details had been entered onto the PAS by admissions staff. Although this safeguarded the validity of the PAS database, it was frustrating for nurses using the care planning system and potentially harmful to the care of patients admitted as emergency cases.

45. There are also problems about which staff are allowed to use the system. Access is often restricted to qualified nurses to ensure that all plans bear an appropriate computer 'signature'. In practice, however, either students are prevented from using the system even under supervision, or passwords are freely revealed. In one case nurses spend more time at the keyboard away from patients and students receive less practice in care planning. In the other it is unclear whether a plan has been produced by a suitably qualified person and confidentiality of patient information could be compromised.

(iii) POOR INDIVIDUALISATION OF PLANNED CARE

46. Computerisation can detract from the individualisation of care plans. Such individualisation is essential to cost-effective patient-centred nursing. It becomes more difficult to involve the patient in drawing up his plan of care. Nurses may have to duplicate their efforts to do this, first producing hand-written notes and then typing the care plan into the computer. Some of the computer systems studied do not provide for entry and audit of review dates for relevant nursing problems and goals. Others automatically insert standard review dates, whether or not these are appropriate for that patient.

47. Attempts to use care planning systems for workload assessment can result in some particularly unhappy compromises and plans which are little more than task lists. Such systems often require all aspects of direct care to be entered into the computer. This generates a mass of unnecessary detail common to many patients on the ward. Not all systems permit entry of free text observations and care goals. Even where it is technically feasible for 'customised units of care' to be created describing special nursing problems, this is frequently discouraged where the plan is used as a basis of workload calculations, because no standard timings can be associated with these interventions. It is sometimes claimed that free text facilities

are unnecessary because nurses can individualise the plan by hand after it has been printed. On the wards studied, there was little evidence of individualisation of printed plans. Also, any annotations that are made are lost whenever plans are reprinted, as they are daily in some hospitals.

48. Some senior nurses believe that there is a temptation to view the computer as an infallible black-box which removes the need for further thought about the patient's needs. It has been claimed that the structure of the more recent menu-driven discourages nurses from giving adequate thought to appropriate interventions and goals for individual patients and inhibits student learning. Such systems typically present the nurse with a list of nursing problems frequently exhibited by the patients cared for on that ward. Having selected appropriate problems, the system invites the nurse to choose from a list of appropriate goals which in turn produces a menu of possible nursing interventions. There is debate as to whether systems which require the nurse to delete inappropriate items are more likely to result in a good care plan than those which require the nurse to select appropriate items.

(iv) SYSTEM HARDWARE CONSTRAINTS

49. At some hospitals, the usefulness of the system is compromised by the configuration of computer hardware on which it is run. Stand alone ward-based systems will require duplicated entry of patient details. It may be more difficult to transfer care plans if patients are moved to another ward. The potential for multi-disciplinary care planning and audit may be more limited if ward terminals are not networked. It may not always be straightforward to transfer selected information to a central machine for quality assurance and research purposes. Equally, where a networked system is reliant on a central processor with limited capacity, it is sometimes only possible to enter or update care plans at specific times. At one hospital studied, it has to be done at night. In such circumstances, the nurse entering the information is unlikely to have adequate knowledge of the patient's condition and progress to be able to plan care appropriately and may have to rely on written notes provided by a nurse from another shift.

A WAY FORWARD

50. Introducing a computer will not solve problems with the quality of care planning overnight. Care planning systems appear to work best on wards which already have good standards of manual care planning, low staff transience, patients with a diversity of problems and fairly rapid throughput. Potential purchasers should therefore consider the ratio of costs to benefits carefully. Assumptions about the way the system would be used should not be over-optimistic. Pilot wards may be more committed to its success than others. It is unlikely to be possible to provide a comparable level of support once the system is extended throughout the hospital.

51. There may be alternative, cheaper ways of improving care planning to meet defined objectives. On some wards a collection of preprinted standardised care plans with spaces for written individualisation might be just as appropriate, particularly if it is not proposed that computerised care planning will form part of a fully integrated NMS. Word-processed plans, calling down standard text as appropriate, may be a realistic option for some longer-stay wards, and one which could be both cheaper and more flexible. Or it might be more beneficial to speed up care planning by providing nurses with dictation facilities and secretarial support. It may be instructive that, despite an emphasis on giving nurses the information that they need to care for patients, none of the French or American hospitals visited has chosen to computerise care planning.

(i) REDUCING THE TIME AND EFFORT REQUIRED TO SET UP SYSTEMS

52. If nevertheless it is decided to opt for computer assisted care planning, for instance as part of an integrated system, it is advisable to choose one that comes with predefined libraries of care. These can be used or modified as desired. Groups of ward nurses should review the care database and the method of compiling and individualising the care plan to ensure that they are suited to the particular needs of patients on their wards. If care planning systems are to be used effectively, it is necessary that ward nurses accept the standards which are implicitly built in to them. But it has been found that, although each ward should have an involvement in selecting the system, there is no need to re-invent the wheel at each new site just to engender a sense of 'ownership'. Documentation should be supplied with the system referencing research supporting the suggested care options so that users can be confident that they are based on a firm scientific rationale. The chosen

system should accommodate all the models of nursing used on the wards and taught by the local College of Nursing. Subsequently the appropriateness of interventions suggested by the computer for patients with specified nursing problems should be periodically reviewed and, if necessary, updated to reflect the latest research findings and nurses' own experience.

(ii) EASY TO USE CARE PLANS

53. Computerised care plans have to meet a number of conflicting objectives. They form a permanent record of each patient's condition, of care planned and actually delivered. They are a care audit tool, a quick reference document, a means of communication and of patient involvement, a plan of work and a strategic plan for management of the patient's stay and discharge. They must be sufficiently concise for a printout to be used during shift handover. A nurse must also be able quickly to look back over the progress of the patient and note important changes since she was last on duty. However they must be forward as well as backward looking. They must show what needs to be done for each individual patient in a way which highlights differences from the care needs of other patients with similar medical conditions. They should help the nurse to plan each patient's care throughout his stay, setting explicit care goals and timescales for achieving them. They should also be easy for other clinicians and patients to read.

54. To cut down unnecessary detail, it should be possible to print selected sections of the plan and to choose either full or abbreviated text. It is helpful for the computer to hold a concise continuation record as well as the complete care plan. Whilst in theory it may be attractive for each plan to embody standards, it is not productive to print for each patient what is, in effect, a full procedure manual whenever a care plan is written or updated. If plans are to be used for subsequent audit, nurses must have time to enter details of care actually given. The system must permit old versions of the plan to be reconstructed, storing details of changes in a way which is economical of space. There must be a clear policy on the length of time after discharge or transfer to another ward for which care plans will remain accessible on the computer. Plans must then be archived in a form which would meet legal requirements should the care provided be challenged subsequently in the courts.

(iii) CAPACITY FOR INDIVIDUALISATION

55. Patient involvement in drawing up and reviewing care plans with nurses must not be lost. Some wards where patients are usually ambulant on admission have found it sufficient for the patient to sit beside the nurse at the computer terminal whilst the care plan is being drawn up. Adequate privacy and an atmosphere conducive to clarification of problems and needs should be provided. One hospital studied had tried maintaining patient involvement by using computer terminals which could be plugged into sockets at the bedside. It will soon be feasible to use hand-held 'notebook' computers to draw up and amend plans. These could later be down-loaded to a networked computer on return to the nursing station.

56. It is advisable to choose a system which facilitates the entry of free text. Care menus should be sufficiently comprehensive, however, to ensure that a minimum of additional text is needed. If the free text facility is to be utilised effectively, nurses will need tuition in basic keyboard skills. And, as argued in 'The Virtue of Patients' more professional development and a change in attitudes will also often be required.

(iv) APPROPRIATE COMPUTER HARDWARE

57. The experience of hospitals who have attempted to introduce computerised care planning 'on the cheap' is not encouraging. Because nursing time is so expensive, it will usually be cost-effective to choose hardware which permits 24 hour access and which minimises duplication of effort in data input. To meet legal requirements and ensure an adequate quality of care, however, nurses must never be prevented by the system from creating or accessing a care plan because it requires prior entry of patient details elsewhere in the hospital.

BETTER USE OF CARE PLANNING SYSTEMS

58. There must therefore be some doubt over the suitability of computer-assisted care planning for many wards. Clarity of thought is essential at the system planning stage about the purpose of the system and the way nurses would use it. Those hospitals which have already installed a system should ensure that:

▼   staff have a proper appreciation of the purpose of care planning and of the contribution that the system can make;

▼ continuing training and support in the use of the system are adequate;

▼ students are able to benefit from the system;

▼ the plans stored on the system present an accurate and complete picture of the care actually delivered;

▼ use of free text to individualise plans is not inhibited:

   (a) by the system itself,

   (b) by policies on the way it is to be used,

   (c) by the attitudes of senior nurses, managers and clinicians,

   (d) by inadequate keyboard skills;

▼ the construction and evaluation of plans includes the patient as a participant in care;

▼ nurses never give the impression that they are more interested in what appears on the computer screen than in talking to patients;

▼ the confidentiality of patient information is not compromised;

▼ plans are being used in the way intended, eg at handover;

▼ the system has resulted in more timely completion of plans, has improved their legibility and has saved nurses' time;

▼ the accuracy and quality of care plans are audited regularly.

Workload Assessment

59. 'The Virtue of Patients' showed that ward staffing varies substantially between hospitals, wards and shifts, often independently of patient needs. Some of this variation is explicable, but much appears to be attributable to poor rostering, to lack of knowledge about nursing workload or inadequate use of the workload information that is available. However, whilst nursing workload assessment can be valuable in improving the efficiency with which this major resource is utilised, the feasibility of accurate and consistent assessment is increasingly being questioned (Ref. 8). This section reviews some of the uncertainties and hidden problems and suggests ways to ensure that workload assessment is used constructively. Manual as well as computerised workload assessment must be considered. The balance of advantages and disadvantages of differing levels of computerisation and networking needs to be carefully weighed (Exhibit 8).

THE POTENTIAL BENEFITS

60. Workload assessment systems offer the prospect of providing data which can be used to improve the match on each shift between available staff and the skills required to meet patient needs and quality of care objectives. Equally importantly, they

Exhibit 8

COMPUTERISING WORKLOAD ASSESSMENT
Advantages and disadvantages of differing levels of computerisation need to be carefully weighed.

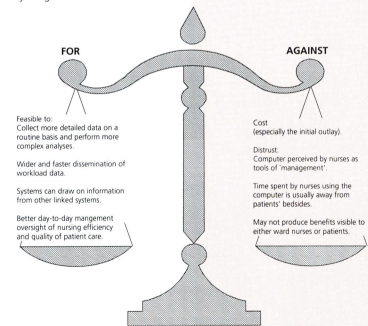

FOR

Feasible to:
Collect more detailed data on a routine basis and perform more complex analyses.

Wider and faster dissemination of workload data.

Systems can draw on information from other linked systems.

Better day-to-day mangement oversight of nursing efficiency and quality of patient care.

AGAINST

Cost
(especially the initial outlay).

Distrust:
Computer perceived by nurses as tools of 'management'.

Time spent by nurses using the computer is usually away from patients' bedsides.

May not produce benefits visible to either ward nurses or patients.

Source: Audit Commission

can help nurses to think about the way in which they organise their work and roster staff and whether this is in tune with patient needs. Would it be appropriate to change the way the work is allocated amongst different grades of staff? Workload information can also be used to help cost the nursing care delivered to specific patients for planning service developments and negotiating contracts. However, such benefits can only be achieved if systems are chosen and used with full knowledge of their individual limitations.

61. Workload systems are often installed primarily to produce information which can be used to review objectively the adequacy of daily ward staffing during the previous month and to inform the setting of establishments. They are particularly suited to this use in settings where there is little movement of nurses between wards. They may either complement or replace 'once-off' establishment-setting methodologies (described in Box C). The advantages of using a system which generates 'continuous' data include:

(i) permitting more objective measurement of workload rather than alignment of staffing with that of other wards;

(ii) showing the range of workload levels with which the ward has to cope as well as the average.

PROBLEMS

(i) DISILLUSIONMENT FLOWING FROM INAPPROPRIATE OBJECTIVES

62. The way in which workload assessment information was actually used at the majority of study sites was disappointing. There was considerable staff disillusionment. This frequently stemmed from over-emphasis on the value of the system as a way in which nurses could provide managers with objective proof of a need for increased ward establishments. When extra staff were not forthcoming, this led to intermittent entry of data which were often also inaccurate. Managers too often lost interest, because systems had not produced the expected staff savings. It was difficult to see how patients had benefited.

63. Hospital managers had often not thought through sufficiently clearly how they intended to use workload information. Assessments can be forward or backward looking (Exhibit 9, overleaf). It is important to be clear which are required since not all systems facilitate both.

Box C

DIFFERING APPROACHES TO SETTING WARD ESTABLISHMENTS

	Top-down Formulae	Consultative approaches	Activity based regression	Bottom-up workload assessment
Examples	(a) Trent (Senior-Gratton), Butts-Milbourne, (b) Some applications of Aberdeen Formula	(a) Telford (1979 -) (b) Brighton (1985)	Teamwork (1987-)	Nursing Management Systems + Criteria for care, GRASP, McGratty, NISCM etc.
HOW	(a) Development (1978-85); Statistical regression techniques were used to relate current hospital nurse staffing levels to (e.g.) number and mix of available beds by speciality, throughput. Application: Strategic planning of new services at hospital level. (b) Development (1967-77): (i) Advisory group defined dependency groups, required basic care and acceptable task frequencies. (ii) Wards meeting these standards chosen as 'models' on which timings were taken (for patients in each dependency group) of basic care, technical care, administrative and miscellaneous tasks. Application can be either: part of a consultative excercise, based on ward acuity for sample period, or as a top-down nurse per available bed formula using regional data for average dependency & occupancy by speciality.	(a) (i) Information gathering:- patient activity/dependency, ward audit of other factors likely to affect staff requirement, current staff availability by shift. (ii) Discussion between ward sister, line manager, independent assessor. Agree/modify desired/minimum staffing and skill mix by time of day suggested by sister. (iii) Convert to w.t.e. establishments: Formulae assume economical shift pattern. Add allowance for leave, sickness, training. (b) (i) Ward sisters record activity and dependency for specifiied periods and acceptable staffing/skill mix for those times. (ii) Convert to establishments (per Telford). (iii) Statistical regression of requested ward establishments against occupied beds/other workload factors to identify 'average' judgement and 'outliers' for further discussion.	Development phase: (i) Nurse in charge of each shift on studied wards recorded number of staff present, quality of care during period, occupied beds, dependency, patient movements, theatre lists etc. (ii) Regression used to determine statistically significant determinants of workload for each type of ward and staffing levels in relation to these, at times when care was judged 'good'. (iii) Application: Agree target quality of care. Substitute activity data for ward into formula to obtain nursing hours required each day. (iv) Add on time required for escorts and meetings, adjust for differing shift lengths, convert to w.t.e staffing.	Each patient's needs for nursing care during each day or shift are assessed. Standard times for different activities or patient groups (based on professional consensus, observation on wards providing good care, or national databases) are applied. Care may be categorised by the grade of staff required. Allowances are added for indirect care and other nursing workload. Hours required are converted into w.t.e staff. Using records of daily staffing requirements over a number of months, decisions can be taken as to what ward establishments, use of temporary staff and overtime would enable demand to be met most efficiently.
PROs:	Quick. Use readily available hard data.	Provide frameworks for exercise of professional judgement which are low cost, transparent, applicable to any sort of ward. Encourage re-examination of ward routines, facilities and resource use. Brighton also provides a formula for strategic planning.	Quick & cheap, using only verifiable data. Consistent results wherever used. Clearly demonstrates the likely effect of varying ward staffing on quality of care. Regular professional quality assessments can be used to check continued formula validity.	Depending on methology, raises staff conciousness of resource usage and review of work patterns. Can predict effect on costs and temporary staff usage of setting establishments to meet differing percentages of peak workload.
CONs:	Reflect historic staffing and patterns of care rather than current need. Insufficiently sensitive for use at ward level. No sense of ownership.	Dependent on local expectations of care standards which themselves reflect historic staffing levels. Ideal staffing shown typically to be 'just one more'.	Little conciousness-raising if applied as a 'black-box' methodology. Assumes quality to be determined by 'pairs of hands' relative to workload and that all work is time-critical. Assessed care quality may be based on standards reflecting historic staffing.	Some are expensive in staff time. If used only to set establishments, nurses become disillusioned with delay & data quality deteriorates. No guarantee of consistency. Methodologies which exclude minimum safety cover/ward overhead can be potentially misleading.

Exhibit 9

WORKLOAD ASSESSMENT

Assessments can be forward or backward looking, analysing past experience or predicting future needs.

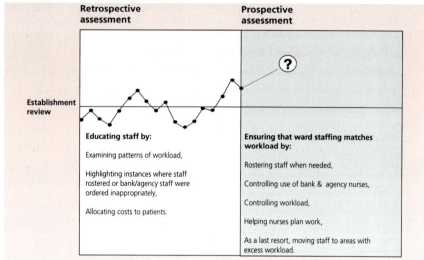

Source: Audit Commission

(a) Difficulties in Matching Staffing to Forecast Workload

64.   Prospective workload assessment systems have often been installed with the assumption that the information produced would be used to move staff from one ward to another for individual shifts or to book additional nurses from banks or agencies in order to even out each nurse's workload. Moving nurses about the hospital in this way negates the potential benefits to continuity of care which could flow from the 'named nurse' standard introduced in the 'Patient's Charter'. Both efficiency and quality of patient care are likely to be reduced if the ward team and its planned disposition are frequently interrupted by temporary transfer of nurses. Imported staff who are not fully familiar with the ward may not know any of the patients or be committed to the ward ethos.

65. There can also be practical difficulties in using systems in this way to match ward staffing with workload on each shift. For instance it may be impossible to project both the occupancy of medical wards and future patient dependency with sufficient certainty to determine future staffing requirements, even for the following day. Only one hospital kept sufficient data for the discrepancy between forecast

and actual workload to be quantified. On the general medical wards studied, nurses' projections of workload for the next 24 hours were extremely inaccurate (Box D, overleaf). There is also insufficient emphasis on the need for timely return and processing of data for nurse managers to have an accurate picture of workload. Delays are often exacerbated by cynicism amongst ward staff that it is more likely that staff will be moved out of the ward than that extra staff will be forthcoming when a deficit is predicted. At many hospitals the system for booking bank or agency staff is not sufficiently responsive to react to short term peaks in workload.

(b) Lack of Constructive Use of Retrospective Data

66. Retrospective workload assessment may be used to educate staff by highlighting instances when there was a mismatch of staffing and assessed workload, or when use of agency and bank staff was not justified by workload. At some sites the approach was not felt to be constructive. It is only useful if the mismatch was predictable and if the ward sister has sufficient short term control over use of temporary staff. Sometimes daily workload assessment data are used only for the occasional review of ward establishments. The accuracy of the assessments suffers if nurses are required to submit data which appear to have no apparent immediate use, each day over a period of years.

67. Other problems can stem from use of inaccurate and systematically biased data. At some hospitals studied, only the forecasts of workload were stored for later retrospective analysis. Later estimates taking account of the numbers of patients actually present and their care needs were seldom entered into the computer. Nurses saw little point in wasting time reassessing patients after the event. This invalidated the data as a means of setting establishments which more accurately reflected workload.

(ii) METHODOLOGICAL DIFFERENCES AND DISAGREEMENTS

68. Many different workload assessment systems are in use. Some studies have found that they can produce estimates of staffing requirements to care for a similar mix of patients which differ by up to 40 per cent, depending on which system is selected, the way in which it is implemented and how its results are interpreted (Ref. 9). Staffing and workload can not be compared even between similar wards in hospitals using the same methodology, since time requirements are often cali-

INACCURATE WORKLOAD PROJECTIONS - A CASE STUDY

The usefulness of workload assessment systems on some wards may be limited by predictive accuracy (Exhibit 10). This case study uses data from two general medical wards that kept both nurses' predictions of the number of staff that would be needed on the following day and retrospective estimates of the actual workload. The system used expresses workload as 'qualified nurse equivalents', unqualified staff counting as the equivalent of different fractions of a nurse depending on their experience. Comparing actual workload on the early and late shifts, shown on the vertical axis of Exhibit 10a, with the predictions:

— on 87% of occasions, nurses underestimated the next day's workload;

— on 20% of shifts this underestimate was greater than 1 qualified nurse equivalent;

The underestimates arose both from the assumptions nurses had been instructed to make about new admissions and from overcautious prediction of patient dependency.

Comparing the actual number of qualified nurse equivalent staff available on the wards with these workload predictions (Exhibit 10b), on 67% of occasions the staffing should have been adequate, although there were large variances between staffing and workload.

These were the results reported to management. However if the actual numbers of staff available are compared with the retrospective estimates of workload (Exhibit 10c), staffing is shown to have been adequate on only 48% of occasions. Management consequently failed to appreciate the true magnitude of the problem. It is therefore essential to monitor workload forecasting accuracy and to ensure that there is an agreed set of data.

Exhibit 10a

ACCURACY OF WORKLOAD PREDICTION ON 2 GENERAL MEDICAL WARDS

Usefulness of workload assessment systems on some wards my be limited by predictive accuracy

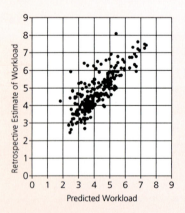

Exhibit 10b

STAFFING VERSUS PREDICTED WORKLOAD ON 2 GENERAL MEDICAL WARDS

More than enough nursing staff were available on most shifts to cover predicted workload

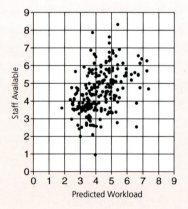

Exhibit 10c

STAFFING VERSUS ACTUAL ASSESSED WORKLOAD ON 2 GENERAL MEDICAL WARDS

...But although enough staff were provided on average, adequacy of cover in relation to actual workload varied even more markedly from shift to shift

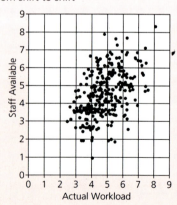

Source: Audit Commission study site (early & late shifts)

brated inconsistently. These differences can only partly be explained by the differing layout and characteristics of each ward.

69. Most *bottom-up* workload methodologies designed for use on a daily or shift basis first require the amounts of nursing time directly needed by each patient to be assessed or calculated. These estimates are then summed and an allowance for nursing duties that do not relate to direct care such as ward administration is added. However, different systems assess both direct care needs and the time needed for indirect care or running the ward in very different ways. This affects both the uses that can be made of the data and their likely acceptability to nurses and managers. Some systems produce estimates of required ward staffing which allow for the minimum levels of cover needed to keep the ward running and maintain patient safety. Others explicitly divorce assessment of workload from such considerations, but may flag up occasions when the staffing required to meet assessed workload would not provide adequate safety cover.

(a) Assessing *Direct Care* Workload – Which approach is 'better'?

70. Methods used to assess direct care requirements[1] can broadly be classified as (a) task based, (b) dependency based, (c) patient activity based, or (d) a mixture of these. These differing approaches with their main advantages and disadvantages are described in Box E, overleaf.

71. There has been much debate as to which approach is 'better'. To some extent, each reflects a distinctive philosophy of nursing. However, no method can be devised that can be proved to be perfectly 'objective'. Each is dependent to some extent on professional judgement, in different ways. Most methodologies require nurses either to place individual patients into dependency categories or to specify the items of care that they should receive. In many, the time allowances for patients

---

1   *One methodology, TEAMWORK, is distinctive amongst those designed for use on a daily or shift by shift basis in that it does not attempt to assess the direct care element of nursing workload separately. Nursing workload is considered as a whole rather than as the aggregate of a number of tasks or of the care needed by individual patients. The formulae used by TEAMWORK do, however, contain some elements which vary according to factors which, although they are not intended to reflect a particular group of tasks, do relate to ward activity and patient needs, and other elements which are constant. For convenience, it is therefore discussed here under the heading of 'patient activity based systems'*

Box E

ASSESSING DIRECT CARE WORKLOAD

	Dependency/ patient need	Systems (patient activity)	Task/nurse activity
Examples	Criteria for Care, NISCM, SENS, McGratty	Teamwork	GRASP, PENFRO, some elements of FIP, (Most integrated systems, CRESCENDO etc., offer a choice of methology; their default options can be considered within this category).
HOW	Each patient is classified, typically according to the level of nursing care needed to support the principal 'activities of daily living' (feeding, mobility, hygiene etc). The average dependency of patients on the ward is known as its 'acuity'. The average times needed to care for patients in each category are established by reference to times taken on one or more 'model wards' for that speciality, judged both to be efficient and providing good quality care. The times required to nurse each patient (expected to be) present are summed.	Development: Nurse in change of each shift on studied wards recorded numbers of staff present, quality of care during that period on a 6 point scale, occupied beds, dependency, movements, theatre lists etc. Regression used to determine what staffing levels in relation to workload indicators produced each level of care on different types of ward. (Dependency proved non-significant statistically)	Direct patient care is divided into a series of nursing tasks and interventions. Each patient's care needs are assessed daily or by shift in terms of these tasks.
			Standard times, frequencies and the grade of staff required are established for each task, using either work study, data from other similar wards, or consensus of professional opinion.
		Application: agree target quality of care, adjust equations for differing shift lengths etc. and insert ward activity levels.	The total time required of each staff category to care for each patient is calculated and summed to give ward workload.
Variants	Time allowances during each shift for other patient needs may be added (for instance a profile of nursing time needed after a patient's return from theatre).	Several forms: strategic planning tool, establishment setting methodology, computerised nursing management system, computer assisted/manual workload information/QA system.	GRASP based systems assess in detail only time required for the 20% most frequent interventions which typically account for 80% of direct care nursing time.
	A broader definition of dependency, embracing the need for nursing time to be devoted to other direct care activities such as patient education, may be adopted. NISCM insists all wards are unique and must develop their own values.	The Oxford system, although very different, also uses 'hard data' about patients and their medical conditions to categorise them into care need groups with agreed standard times based on historic care plans.	FIP based systems use dependency to assess time needed for basic patient care and task lists for more specialised interventions.
Integration with care plans	Dependency may be assessed directly from care plans (this is claimed to be more objective than if a nurse makes a separate assessment).	None.	Some integrated systems generate lists of required tasks and interventions directly from care plans. As an alternative to direct use of standard times, planned care can be compared with that delivered by known staff levels on previous days. Other systems use task lists to generate an outline care plan.
PROs	Consistent with nursing philosophy of holistic care. Recognises that nurses do more than one thing at a time.	Only easily collected 'hard' data are used. Provides a record of nurses' assessments of quality of care provided on each shift, related to staffing and skill mix.	A more intuitively obvious breakdown of what nurses do and how long it takes. More explicit assumptions facilitate validity/consistency audit.
CONs	Variable consistency and objectivity of classification. Assumes quality of care can be replicated with a given level of staffing relative to patient dependency or need. Strict use of dependency underestimates need for psychological care /rehabilitation.	'Black box' methodology - has little conciousness-raising value. The basic Teamwork system assumes levels of care to be determined primarily by availability of 'pairs of hands', but correlation between quality and staffing on individual shifts appears poor.	Could encourage 'task based' thinking. Problems where activities are carried out in parallel. Accuracy of standard timings often low.

in the various dependency categories or for the specified nursing tasks are set by nurses, as are the assumptions about what proportion of their time should be spent directly caring for patients. Even systems such as *TEAMWORK* which produce assessments based on 'hard' statistical data use formulae which depend on nursing assessments of the quality of care provided. Thus ward nursing workload assessment and establishment setting systems can only usefully suggest *relative* levels and mixes of staffing needed on 'similar' wards, or at different times.

72. Despite the effort put into development of workload methodologies, there must be some doubts as to their statistical robustness. A number of aspects of the validity of different systems in discriminating appropriately between the care needs of different patients and of the reliability with which they are used may be considered (Exhibit 11, Ref. 10). For example, there can be considerable variance in the time

Exhibit 11

THE VALIDITY AND RELIABILITY OF WORKLOAD ASSESSMENT METHODOLOGIES

A number of aspects of the validity of different systems in discriminating appropriately between the care needs of different patients and of the reliability with which they are used may be considered

Does the way that the system discriminates between the needs of different patients match:	**Validity**	**Reliability**	Are workload assessments consistent:
The hospital's nursing philosophy?	**Construct Validity**	**Intra-rater Reliability**	When the same nurse assesses patients with similar needs. or later reassesses a stable patient?
Critical need factors?	**Content Validity**		
Nurses' own perceptions of patients' care needs?	**Face Validity**	**Inter-rater Reliability**	When a number of nurses assess the same patient?
Nurses' current behaviour?	**Concurrent Validity**	**Inter-system Reliability**	...And would similar conclusions be drawn if the same assessments were processed at different hospitals, or using another system?
...And can it produce accurate forecasts?	**Predictive Validity**		

Source: Audit Commission

3 Workload Assessment

Exhibit 12

NON-DIRECT -CARE WORKLOAD

Workload caused by duties other than direct patient care is either assumed to be proportional to direct care needs, or is calculated in a variety of different ways.

METHODOLOGY A

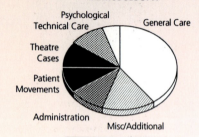

- Psychological Technical Care
- General Care
- Theatre Cases
- Patient Movements
- Administration
- Misc/Additional

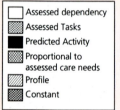

Legend:
- Assessed dependency
- Assessed Tasks
- Predicted Activity
- Proportional to assessed care needs
- Profile
- Constant

METHODOLOGY B

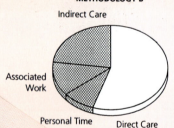

- Indirect Care
- Associated Work
- Personal Time
- Direct Care

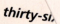

needed either to perform the same set of nursing interventions or to provide adequate care to patients in the same dependency category. The magnitude of such differences can be greater than that between time allowances for different categories of patients (Ref. 11) or between different interventions. Staffing levels alone do not appear to be a good predictor of the quality of care provided with a particular mix of patients on an individual shift. Replication of staffing levels in relation to patient needs does not necessarily produce the same quality of nursing care. There are many ways in which care can be improved without additional nursing resources.

73. Systems which assess workload directly from care plans have been particularly problematic. None of the UK hospitals studied had managed to produce acceptable assessments in this way. This is mainly because so many of the nursing interventions specified can be carried out in parallel. Nurses may be assessing, planning and delivering care to patients all at the same time. Other interventions require more than one nurse. Systems which allow workload assessment data to be entered alongside care plans, rather than generating them automatically, can be more successful.

(b) Indirect care and ward overheads

74. Activity studies show that direct patient care typically accounts for only about a half of the nurse's workload, although there are some differences between systems in how this is defined. Whichever method is used to measure this direct care workload, allowances and overheads have to be added for indirect or shared care, ward administration and 'personal time'. Workload caused by nurses' other duties is variously assumed to be proportional to direct care needs, to the number of occupied beds, a constant independent of ward size and occupancy, or distributed according to predefined daily and shift patterns (Exhibit 12). This is a comparatively under-researched area. It can not be assumed that on each shift total workload will be proportional to direct patient care needs, or even that the overhead will remain constant. Yet there is little point in measuring direct care workload to the minute (one system claims even greater precision) if there is no objective basis for the assessment of other work which is often almost half of the total workload.

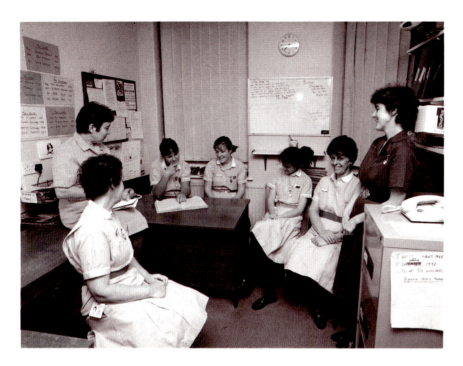

Exhibit 12 (continued)

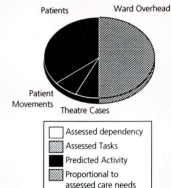

METHODOLOGY C

Patients — Ward Overhead

Patient Movements — Theatre Cases

- Assessed dependency
- Assessed Tasks
- Predicted Activity
- Proportional to assessed care needs
- Profile
- Constant

METHODOLOGY D

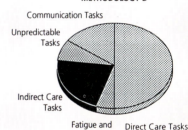

Communication Tasks

Unpredictable Tasks

Indirect Care Tasks

Fatigue and Delay

Direct Care Tasks

75. Nor is it straightforward to decide which form of assumption about overheads is 'correct'. Not all nursing work is time-critical. Some patient care must be given immediately on demand or at a set time. There are fixed times too for such activities as handovers and meetings elsewhere in the hospital. But nurses have some discretion as to when during the day they bathe a patient, teach a student, or update care plans. It may not be too disastrous if some planned activity is occasionally omitted or postponed. Some administrative activities can be deferred for a number of days if the ward is busy or brought forward if it is slack – the so called *push-pull* workload effect. Naturally, there are limits to the length of time for which a significant proportion of workload can be postponed. Another complication is that the proportion of work which is time-critical would appear to vary by type of patient, by grade of staff and by time of day. Also, like the rest of us, many nurses work faster when they are busy. The length of time for which they can keep this up without deterioration in quality of care must depend on the individual, on training and on the state of morale in the ward.

76. The treatment of non-direct care matters because it determines the extent to which workload assessments can reliably be used without modification to compare the adequacy of staffing between wards. It is also a significant factor in the way staff requirements are assumed to vary as direct care workload changes with occupancy and patient needs (Exhibit 13). If, for example, information on predicted workload is used to cost contracts that would involve major changes to activity levels, or to assess what reductions could be made to ward staffing if beds were to be closed, misleading conclusions may be drawn if the assumptions made about non-direct care are 'inappropriate'.

77. The need for a constant ward overhead is intuitively appealing as there seems no obvious reason to assume, as do a number of workload methodologies, that for

Exhibit 13

ALTERNATIVE APPROACHES TO INCLUSION OF WARD OVERHEAD
The treatment of non-direct care is significant in determining the way staff requirements are assumed to vary as direct care workload changes with patient needs.

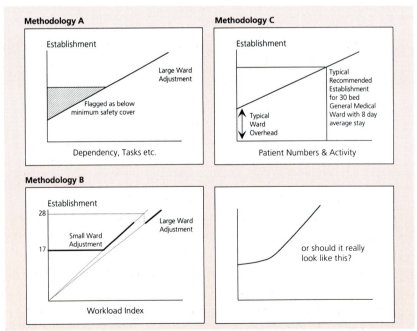

Source: Audit Commission

example ward administration and meetings take longer at times when the average dependency of patients on the ward is higher. Against this, it can be argued that more time could be needed in these circumstances for some non-direct care, for instance completion of care plans, ward rounds and handovers.

78. North West Region's *Teamwork* study (Ref. 12) attempted to resolve this by examining the way in which nurses' assessments of quality of care on each shift varied in relation to staffing and workload indicators. It used statistical regression techniques to produce ward staffing equations which suggest that about half of the nursing workload on a typical general medical ward is an overhead, independent of the number or care needs of patients present. Its findings are not conclusive, since the approach adopted did not attempt to distinguish between workload overheads and minimum safety cover. They could also have been affected by the degree of *push-pull* operating on the studied wards. Care may have been rated as 'good' at times when staffing was below the average required for that level of workload, simply because some non patient-related activities were being postponed. These factors may help to reconcile *Teamwork's* findings with the apparently contradictory conclusions of the research underlying *Criteria for Care* that, over the *longer* term, total nursing workload *can* be assumed to be proportional to direct care. Current work to refine *Teamwork's* quality measure by ascertaining what kinds of work are omitted or postponed when staffing falls below that required for good care will help to throw more light on this question.

(c) Skill mix requirements

79. Skill mix reviews have traditionally been based either on consultative exercises or on activity analyses. The latter (e.g. Ref. 13) require ward activities to be classified according to whether they should be undertaken by a nurse, or could be carried out by a care assistant or other types of staff. Such studies can only provide a rough guide to the average mix of skills required on the ward. The decision as to who should, for example, give a bed bath should be influenced as much by the condition of the individual patient on that day as by the degree of skill required by the physical task. A qualified nurse may use this time to provide support or information to patients, or to encourage their rehabilitation. Nurses can use their experience to estimate the average proportion of occasions on which it is appropriate to delegate such duties. But on some shifts in acute wards there will be

insufficient work to occupy a care assistant. On others it would be necessary to adopt a very task oriented approach to care to keep her occupied. Unfortunately many of the more routine duties suitable for delegation must be performed on demand and can not be postponed until someone of the 'right' grade is available. The final decision on skill mix must therefore remain with the ward sister. Greater credence than warranted is sometimes given to the results of seemingly objective studies.

(iii) INEFFICIENT OR INAPPROPRIATE OPERATION

80. Patient dependency or care requirements are sometimes assessed by nurses with insufficient knowledge of the patient. This usually happens either because the number of nurses who are allowed or trained to use the system is unduly restricted, or because the computer can only be used for workload assessment at certain times of the day or night. For similar reasons, at some other hospitals, workload data are transcribed from manually completed sheets into the computer by qualified nurses. This is clearly an inappropriate use of nurses' time. At some, they had to leave the ward to use the computer because the only terminals were located elsewhere in the hospital. Since other duties took priority, nurses were unable to access data quickly and up-to-date information was often unavailable. They typically perceived the system as being solely for the benefit of management and made little use of it themselves.

WORKLOAD ASSESSMENT - A WAY FORWARD
(i) MORE APPROPRIATE USE

81. The value of workload assessment systems is that they encourage nurses and management to:

▼　　define the quality of service that they should be providing;

▼　　consider the relative levels of ward resources needed from day to day to reflect changing patient needs and other workload;

▼　　examine patterns of workload, so helping ward sisters to roster staff more appropriately or to change their working patterns so as to make better use of available staff;

▼ ensure that bank and agency staff are used at times of staff shortage only when justified by projected workload;

▼ examine the need for specific nursing activities critically with respect to the contribution which they make to the quality of care delivered to the patient;

▼ organise these activities in an efficient, coherent and cohesive manner;

▼ regulate, where possible, the mix of patients admitted to wards and consequent nursing workload so as to ensure that an acceptable level of care can be provided within available nurse resources;

▼ consider quantified data when negotiating ward establishments and reviewing skill mix.

82. In exceptional circumstances, a workload assessment system may need to be used to help nurses decide which staff can be released to help out other wards without major detriment to patient care. But this should not be the prime purpose for collection of workload information. It is important too that ward sisters are fully involved in such day to day decisions about staff movements and that these are not determined mechanistically. Proper management training for ward sisters and devolution of pay and budgets for employment of bank and agency staff to wards is essential if such decisions are to be taken on a rational but sensitive basis.

83. If more effective use is to be made of prospective workload projections, forecasting accuracy must be monitored and if necessary improved. A number of hospitals have investigated workload determinants, seasonal and weekly workload patterns. Some hospitals could make more use of information on impending discharges. Good information on impending admissions may never be possible for wards with a high proportion of emergency admissions. But details of patients elsewhere in the hospital awaiting transfer to the ward could usefully be incorporated. Realistic estimates of potential first day care needs should be included for possible admissions. Both optimistic and pessimistic estimates of workload based on alternative scenarios could be produced.

84. Greater emphasis on timely return and processing of data may be required. This should be reinforced by demonstration that effective action will be taken to

restrict workload in the interests of patients or to provide additional staff when the system shows that there is likely to be a severe shortage of nurses over a sustained period. It must also be made clear that wards that are run efficiently will not be penalised by temporary transfer of nurses in circumstances where this would be detrimental to continuity of care.

85. The system used to book bank and agency nurses needs overhaul in many hospitals. Devolving more responsibility for this to wards should secure a faster and more appropriate response to forecast needs. As noted in 'The Virtue of Patients', a number of hospitals have improved the cohesiveness of ward staffing by restricting employment of individual bank nurses to a small number of wards with which they are familiar and ensuring that they can be booked or cancelled at short notice. Others are encouraging more use of overtime to cover short periods of peak workload rather than increasing establishments or employing bank staff for a full shift. Workload assessment is essential for such decisions and to ensure that arrangements to supplement staffing work effectively.

(ii) PUTTING METHODOLOGICAL DIFFERENCES INTO PERSPECTIVE

86. Nearly all of the available systems, regardless of methodology, could if used appropriately lead to some improvement in nursing productivity and more consistency in standards of patient care. They can alert the nurse in charge to forthcoming shifts on which it is likely that work will need to be re-ordered. They can give early warning of periods when extra help will be needed so that nurses have enough time to plan how additional staff can be utilised in ways which minimise disruption to continuity of care for patients. They can be used to inform decisions taken when patients are admitted about which nurse or team of nurses will be best placed to care for them during their stay and how other workload should be divided amongst nurses. This helps to ensure consistency with the preferred method of organising care. Also, in a stable environment, their assessments should be sufficiently accurate for costing the care delivered to patients.

87. Most *bottom-up* workload assessment methodologies have the beneficial effect during their implementation phase of getting nurses to think about the way in which they do their job, heightening awareness of the way time is used and of quality issues. But some (eg the *NISCM* system) place greater emphasis on continuing this

conciousness-raising once the system is operational. Because the perceived 'owner-ship' of the system by the ward is seen to be so important for this to occur, a trade off has to be made between such benefits and estimation of workload in a way which is demonstrably consistent with other wards. A decision needs to be taken at the outset as to the right balance of objectives at the present time. Managers, doctors, other clinicians and nurses need a common understanding of the limitations of each methodology as well as its strengths, if installed systems are not to produce a mass of data with little practical impact. The project team, together with representative nurses and managers should simulate the way they see the system and the information it will produce being used before the Statement of Need is finalised. The exceptional circumstances under which action would be taken to limit nursing workload should be agreed between ward sisters, senior nurses, managers and clinicians at the outset. Such action might involve bed closures or rescheduling admission to increase the proportion of patients that are less dependent on nursing care. Guidelines should also be agreed for the circumstances in which nurses would be transferred, overtime or use of temporary staff authorised.

88. **Skill Mix:** The traditional consultative and activity analysis approaches remain a valuable way to focus thought about skill mix requirements. They are a useful way to identify additional clerical and housekeeping duties that should not be undertaken by nurses at times when they could economically be performed by less skilled staff. They can inform discussion of the appropriate role and need for care assistants. However, decisions should take into account the timing of patient needs, the way care is organised on the ward and the effects of any planned moves towards primary nursing.

89. A new 'systems' approach, recently piloted by nurses in North West Region and the York Health Economics Consortium (Ref. 14), may soon offer an alternative. Indicators based on whether nurses provided specific types of care and undertook their other duties within acceptable time scales were first defined. It was found to be possible to combine these indicators in a way which would predict nurses' judgements about the quality of care provided on individual shifts. An experiment was undertaken to show how the indicators changed when the numbers of 'pairs of hands' and the skill mix were varied. It suggested that, on the types of ward and within the limited range of variation tested, quality of care could be

Exhibit 14

SKILL MIX EXPERIMENT (NORTH WESTERN RHA)
Quality of Care could be improved without increasing costs by reducing the number of staff and increasing the skill-mix

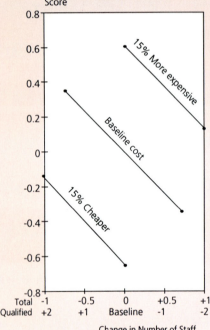

Change in Teamwork "Care Level" Score

- 15% More expensive
- Baseline cost
- 15% Cheaper

| Total | -1 | -0.5 | 0 | +0.5 | +1 |
| Qualified | +2 | +1 | Baseline | -1 | -2 |

Change in Number of Staff
(Baseline: 3 qualified 2 others)

Note: *The lines show combinations with approximately equal staffing costs*

Source: *Based on the findings of North West RHA/York Health Economics Consortium Skill Mix Study*

improved without increasing costs by reducing the number of staff and increasing the skill mix (Exhibit 14). These results accord with the professional judgement of many nurses (e.g. Refs. 15 – 17) including most of those interviewed by the Audit Commission. One explanation offered is that qualified nurses can order their work more flexibly to meet patient needs and do not have to wait for instructions or for a suitable task. It is to be hoped that this experimental approach will rapidly be developed into a skill-mix methodology usable on wards of varying specialties.

(iii) EFFICIENT ENTRY OF DATA

90. Where shared computer terminals remote from the ward are still in use, data should be entered by ward clerks or other clerical staff rather than by nurses. However with the continuing decline in costs of computer equipment, it could now be economic to replace these with ward based terminals. If these could not be networked, 'floppy disks' could be used to transfer information to a central computer for later analysis.

REVIEWING EXISTING WORKLOAD ASSESSMENT SYSTEMS

91. Reviews should encompass:

▼ The reliability of the patient classification methodology.

Does the system discriminate between the time needed to care for differing patients in a way which is consistent with the ward's philosophy of care, the hospital's nursing strategy, nurses' own views of the holistic care needs of each patient and the ways in which they actually prioritise their time? Staff questionnaires, discussion groups and expert review panels may be used to establish this. Timings of care delivered to each patient interpreted in conjunction with assessments of duties or interventions that had to be omitted or postponed may be useful in validating conclusions.

▼ The adequacy of procedures for ensuring that patient care needs are assessed consistently.

▼ The accuracy of workload predictions and ways in which it could be improved.

▼ The timeliness of information and of consequent action.

▼ The extent to which workload information has been used to review ward establishments or skill mix.

▼ Whether the uses made of workload information are compatible with maximising continuity of patient care. Have clear ground-rules been agreed?

▼ Has workload information resulted in any savings in the cost of temporary staff? Could stand-by rostering or ward banks be used to make numbers of staff on duty more responsive to variations in patient need without sacrificing continuity of care?

▼ Do nurses actually make use of the information when prioritising and planning their workload so as best to meet patient needs?

▼ Is the information presented in the most helpful way?

▼ Is additional training, education or support needed?

▼ The efficiency of data entry procedures.

▼ System security and equipment reliability.

4

Rostering

92.   'Rostering' is perhaps a misnomer. Most of the computerised rostering packages currently available offer a range of personnel management features built around the central functions of creating, monitoring and costing *off-duties*. The actual rostering process may be automatic, or based on a pre-specified *'template'* roster, or manual. Fully automatic systems, eg those referred to as employing *'turbo-rostering'*, use a set of algorithms and constraints prespecified by the project nurse in consultation with the ward sisters. A record of agreed leave, requests for time off or shift preferences is also kept on the computer and is taken into consideration when it produces a draft roster. Some systems can be linked to prospective workload assessments. If staff requirements can be predicted far enough in advance, this makes it easier to schedule an appropriate number and mix of nurses on each shift and to flag up deficiencies. *'Template'* rostering systems are based on a user specified standard cyclical roster which is rolled forward each period and reconciled with staff *requests*. Simpler systems require entry of a manually compiled draft roster onto a computer spreadsheet. The computer costs it, produces shift totals and checks the number of hours to be worked by each nurse during the period. If roster data are only required for costing care or analysing time-out, it may be entered retrospectively.

THE POTENTIAL BENEFITS OF COMPUTERISATION

93. Users gave four main reasons for installing a computerised ward nursing rostering system:

(i)   the potential time saving time for the person drawing up the *off-duty*,

(ii)   production of better, clearer rosters that can be easily and accurately updated,

(iii)   more efficient completion and analysis of staffing and time-out returns,

    (iv) more realistic costing of the nursing care actually provided to specific groups of patients.

94. Systems were often perceived to have successfully met these objectives, particularly in hospitals where nurse rostering has traditionally been controlled centrally. However such success is unlikely to be sustainable in the face of the move towards primary nursing and its added emphasis on ensuring continuity of patient care. The main benefits of existing computerised rostering systems in the longer term may flow from their costing and personnel features. Further development is needed before they can be used to help ward sisters roster nurses in ways which improve continuity of care and make more efficient use of their staff for the benefit of patients.

PROBLEMS
(i) FAILURE TO REALISE THE ANTICIPATED TIME SAVINGs

95. At many hospitals, time savings in producing the *off-duty* have been found to be the least successful and useful feature of rostering systems. Those nurses who formerly spent a long time compiling the roster almost invariably did so in their own time. This must be taken into consideration when the potential benefit of releasing time for other duties is estimated since, once computerised, the *off-duty* has to be produced in working hours. On a number of the wards studied, a roster is first drawn up manually and then simply typed into the computer. Not only on these wards do nurses spend more rather than less time on rostering, but the potential for confusion is also increased. The written draft may continue to be used as a working roster. Instances were noted when not all subsequent amendments were entered both into the computer and onto the written copy. This resulted in confusion and occasionally missed shifts.

96. On wards where less emphasis is placed on the need to promote continuity of care by achieving balanced teams on each shift, a roster can be drawn up manually in less than half an hour. The potential for time savings in such cases is consequently small. Computerisation may actually slow down production of the roster. At a number of hospitals there were complaints that time consuming duplicated entry of data, for instance names of student nurses allocated to the ward, was

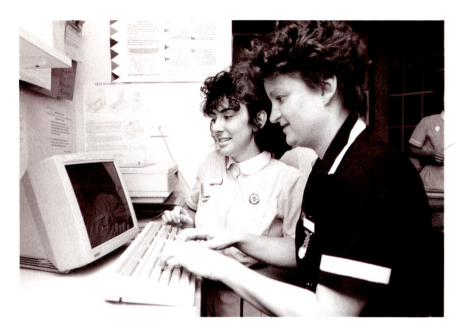

required because there was no link between the rostering system and other hospital computer systems.

97. Anticipated time savings from automated completion of payroll and other returns can also prove elusive. Despite the security and data validation features built into many packages, none of the hospitals studied had reached agreement on using information from rostering systems for direct input to payroll systems. Little use was observed of analyses of absence levels and patterns.

(ii) BETTER ROSTERS NOT GUARANTEED.

(a) Difficulties in rostering by team

98. If a ward is organised in teams, a good roster requires that each team has adequate cover of an appropriate skill mix on every daytime shift. It may be necessary to ensure that the team leader is rostered 'on' when consultant rounds are to take place and that skill mix is higher when the ward is on emergency take. Similar, but more complex, considerations apply when 'primary nursing' has been introduced. Increasingly therefore, ward rosters are built up by combining a number of separate drafts prepared by each primary nurse or team leader. This helps to

improve continuity of care and ensures that cover is arranged by the nurses who know the needs of their patients best. But none of the leading systems will *automatically* roster nurses by team or primary nursing group unless each is set up as if it were a separate ward. If this is done, teams are rostered completely separately with no allowance for interchange of auxiliaries or other nurses. Most of the available systems do not even permit the display of rosters by team so that the balance of cover can be easily checked.

(b) Disappointment with automatic rostering capabilities.

99. Even on wards that roster staff more traditionally, there has been disappointment with the automatic rostering capabilities of some of the more sophisticated systems. Many of those currently available were written initially for the US market. There have been teething troubles, both with terminology and in adapting them to the kinds of staffing levels and shift patterns worked in British hospitals. At one study site, sisters rejected a system introduced to the wards because it was unable to produce a roster with the number of staff available to them. It has proved difficult for users to build into the rostering algorithms traditional conventions such as a 'late' shift following an 'off' so that nurses get the benefit of a full handover, preferences for an early duty before a day off, and students rostered on the same shifts as their 'mentors' wherever possible.

(c) Misleading shift totals

100. A less obvious problem is that some systems print incorrect totals for the numbers of nurses rostered on duty at various times of day. Whilst this may be a relatively trivial problem, it is a further source of potential confusion for ward sisters and managers trying to check that cover is adequate. The 'error' occurs because the programs have been designed primarily to cost the roster. They calculate cover as a by-product of this costing process, by dividing the number of hours worked within specified time bands by the durations of these bands. This works well in most U.S. hospitals, but not for British wards with afternoon shift overlaps, part time nurses and a wide range of overlapping shifts.

101. Putting off-duties onto a computer ought to open the door to analysis of the extent to which desired staffing levels are being achieved and whether it is possible to organise care in the way intended by the ward sister. However, the statistics

offered by existing rostering packages are geared mainly towards payroll, staff costing, analyses of absence patterns and reasons for lost time. Programs should be available to help nurses improve the continuity of patient care within current staffing budgets, but at present these have to be custom written.

A WAY FORWARD

(i) THE RIGHT TARGET FOR TIME SAVINGS

102. Computerised rostering systems can be worthwhile, but have often been found to be of more use to nurse managers, than to ward sisters. They provide a quick source of reference to how many and which nurses are expected to be on duty at any one time. Potential gaps in coverage, especially at night, can be more easily spotted and remedied in good time by suggesting a change of shifts, ordering bank or agency nurses, or, if essential, negotiating the loan of a nurse to another ward. Some nurse managers use reports from rostering systems to check that planned off-duties make economical use of staff and that duties have been divided equitably amongst nurses. 'Time out' information is used both to keep track of staff development and to systematically analyse reasons for absence.

103. The major rostering systems also provide a handy and flexible nursing personnel database. Although this was the feature most valued by nurse managers at the hospitals studied, careful consideration should be given as to whether such use should be encouraged. Much of this information is likely to duplicate that on hospitals' main personnel systems. Whilst this is both wasteful and a potential source of confusion, rostering packages currently offer quicker access to information and give nurses control over the quality of data stored. They can be used to store more specialised information such as nurses' professional registration expiry dates and can save nurse managers much time in compiling ad-hoc returns. They also help if, in an emergency, it is necessary to locate quickly a nurse who speaks a particular language or has a particular skill.

(ii) IMPROVING THE QUALITY OF ROSTERING

(a) An overview of rosters

104. Systems need to be able to cope with the demands of primary and team nursing and to produce rosters which support continuity of care for patients. Currently available fully automatic rostering programs are less suitable for this than simpler

systems. More sophisticated systems are also less likely to justify their costs if rosters are built up by team. However, regardless of how 'off-duties' are initially compiled, a computerised facility for recording rosters can still be of value. If the nurse in charge is reliant on paper rosters, it can be difficult for her to get an authoritative overall picture of who is available and who worked when, particularly where a large number of different or flexible shifts are worked. A computerised system is particularly useful if an on-call arrangement has been introduced whereby nurses nominate additional or alternative shifts that they could work if necessary.

(b) Realistic expectations of automated rostering

105. For automated rostering to be effective, adequate information on factors that might upset workload predictions must be received by the ward. Procedures may need to be reviewed. Examples of such factors include cancelled theatre sessions or changes in case mix likely to result from surgeons' holiday plans. It is wise too before purchase to require suppliers to demonstrate that their products can produce a roster from actual historic staff availability data for one of the more hard pressed wards in the hospital. The practicality of the resulting *off-duty* should be reviewed with the ward sister. However, use of automated rostering packages is only ever likely to prove beneficial in settings where cyclical variations in nursing workload can be predicted with reasonable accuracy some time in advance and where the care needs of the type of patients treated make physical continuity of care a less important consideration. In other circumstances, it may be better to opt for a simpler form of computer assisted system such as one based on 'templates'.

(c) Analysing rosters to improve their quality

106. Rostering packages employ a mass of valuable data on planned and actual ward staffing, including temporary nurses employed on the ward. These could be used to produce graphs, exception reports and summary indicators showing periods when cover was inadequate either in total or, if relevant, by team or primary nursing group, patterns of staffing and costs, the stability of staffing on the ward. An example of such an analysis carried out by the Audit Commission is described in Box F.

Box F

ANALYSING OFF-DUTIES USING DATA FROM COMPUTERISED ROSTER PACKAGES

An analysis of off-duties was conducted on a ward practising team nursing. Rosters were amended to show periods when bank or borrowed staff had been assigned to the ward. A high proportion of part-shifts were worked so the shift totals shown on the roster were sometimes misleading. For the purpose of the analysis, each period of the day, bounded by times when nurses came on or went off duty, was considered separately. A summary indicator of grade mix was used to examine the 'richness' of staffing present at different times. This was calculated by summing the total basic salary cost at grade midpoints of staff present on the ward and dividing the result by the cost of the same number of grade D nurses. The following exception reports, tables and graphs were produced:

(a) Exception reports:

— periods when the minimum safe cover specified by the ward sister was not available;

— periods when the number of qualified nurses present fell below a specified level;

— periods when the most senior nurse on duty was graded below 'E';

— for each team, daytime periods when no nurses from that team were on duty;

— periods when one team was left uncovered by its own nurses, but some other teams had more than the minimum level of staffing;

— periods when the number of staff present exceeded the normal maximum requirement for more than a specified length of time;

— periods when the summary grade mix indicator fell outside a predetermined band of values;

— nurses who worked an abnormally high or low number of weekend duties.

   (Cover was also examined in relation to predicted workload.)

(b) Tables including:

— 24 hour cost of staffing the ward each day (including supplementary duty payments), tabulated by day of week.

(c) Graphs:

— average numbers of qualified and total staffing by period of day;

— average values of the grade mix indicator by time of day and day of week;

— histogram showing distribution of daily staff costs;

— histograms of numbers of staff present by day at particular times of the morning and afternoon;

— scatter plot of actual staff rostered versus predicted workload.

(d) Summary indicators showing the extent to which the planned organisation of care and continuity of care could be maintained within the rosters analysed:

— stability of staffing from day to day: the number of *different* nurses employed on the ward (during the period studied) to provide cover equivalent to one full time nurse; this figure is high if large numbers of different bank or other temporary staff are used, lower if only permanent staff or temporary staff familiar with the ward and its patients are employed);

— the average number of consecutive days for which each nurse was on duty (calculated separately for qualified nurses, all permanent ward staff and all staff who worked on the ward); this shows the number of days for which a short stay patient could expect to have the same nurse looking after him;

— the proportion of the time that students worked on the ward for which their mentor was also on duty.

On this occasion, it was not possible to compare planned with actual rosters to analyse the reasons for differences and for the use of temporary staff.

Findings:

On the ward studied, teams were often imbalanced with several nurses present from one team and none from another. Off duties were not consistent with the chosen model of organisation of care. This was likely to be detrimental to continuity of patient care.

There were two periods in the day (in addition to meal breaks) when, because of the number of nurses working part shifts, the ward was often left in the charge of a D grade nurse.

The cost of staffing the ward from day to day varied by a factor of two to one. There was no correlation between rostered staffing and predicted workload.

A large number of bank staff were used. There was little consistency in the allocation of temporary staff to wards from day to day. 8.6 *different* staff were used to provide the equivalent number of hours of care to one full time permanent member of staff.

Students seldom worked the same shifts as their mentors.

5

Implementation & evaluation

107. Section 1 discussed the assessment of current practices in relation to the chosen nursing strategy and the decisions to be made about which of the problems identified can be addressed through better information. Sections 2 to 4 drew attention to some of the pitfalls that can occur with each of the principal nursing management system functions, together with the ways in which they can be avoided. This section discusses the prerequisites for effective use of a nursing system.

PROBLEMS

(i) LACK OF COMMITMENT AND INVOLVEMENT

108. There was little enthusiasm amongst nurses for the majority of the computerised systems that had been tried out or implemented on the wards studied. A common theme, reported also by Keen and Malby (Ref. 7), was that systems had resulted in additional work for qualified nurses with little proven benefit for the patient. They were perceived to be of little value to those required to operate them, whilst they saw no evidence of constructive use by managers of the data which they entered. The pace and timing of system implementation was often seen as having been poorly co-ordinated with that of other change on the wards. In consequence it was seen as just one more burden imposed on nurses by management.

109. Although efforts had been made to engender a sense of ownership by involving interested ward nurses in system implementation, this was typically a one off effort. There was a feeling that nurses had been involved in specifying the detail of the system, but not in discussing the way in which it should be used. It was often only the minority of enthusiasts who were genuinely committed to use of the system. Problems arose when these nurses moved on.

(ii) INSUFFICIENT EDUCATION AND SUPPORT

110.   The need for adequate initial and continuing training and support from the project team has frequently been underestimated. Tuition may need to be tailored to quite a low level of initial understanding. A recent survey (Ref. 18) found that only 23 per cent of qualified nurses claimed to know what a nursing information system was. However, many of the nurses interviewed felt that they had only been shown the basics of how to input data to the system. Little advice was available on how to explore its full potential and use the computer to examine their practice.

(iii) INAPPROPRIATE COSTING OF PATIENT CARE

111.   A major stated objective of some installed nursing management systems is to provide data which can be used to cost the care delivered to individual patients or specific types of patient. This would facilitate contract costing and consideration of the resource implications of changing case mix or capacity. However none of the hospitals studied was yet using information from workload and rostering systems for such purposes. Evidence that diagnosis related groups or other common case mix indicators are significant discriminators of nursing costs is as yet slight. It is also necessary to make heroic assumptions when attributing the costs of indirect care and other ward staffing overheads to individual patients. It does not seem to be universally appreciated that nursing costs should be calculated differently depending on the purposes for which the data are to be used. For instance, it may be appropriate to cost either average or marginal workload.

(iv) LACK OF EVALUATION

112.   None of the hospitals studied had conducted a full evaluation of the costs and benefits of continuing to operate a nursing management system. Evaluations, where undertaken, have typically been confined to such areas as changes in nursing shift patterns following activity analyses undertaken during the implementation of workload assessment systems. Project nurses at a number of the sites studied reviewed data accuracy periodically. Several had instituted reviews of training and support needs. Management at one hospital had changed their system strategy following a review of whether that originally specified could provide the required information. But broad evaluations of the effects on delivery of patient care appear to be rare (Ref. 19).

SUCCESSFUL IMPLEMENTATION
(i) SECURING COMMITMENT

113. Successful implementation depends heavily on setting the right system objectives and communicating them, clearly and consistently, to nurses, clinicians and managers. Adequate time for broad consultation must therefore be allowed at the planning stage. One hospital visited admitted that it is almost impossible to pick the right moment for consultation. If it is left too late, staff feel that decisions have been taken over their heads. If it takes place too early there is more room for misunderstanding. On balance it was felt right to involve all relevant staff from the start and give them the chance to contribute ideas. The 'Step by Step Guide' similarly suggests that a 'Staff Appreciation Day' is held early on. But until plans are sufficiently advanced, it is advisable to emphasise that introduction of computerised systems is only one possible way forward.

114. Senior managers should demonstrate their commitment to implementing change. They should beware of raising false expectations of changes that are likely to follow implementation of an NMS, whether they be of de-skilling or of substantially increased ward establishments. Such misconceptions, once aroused, can hinder the successful use of any system that may eventually be implemented. Ward

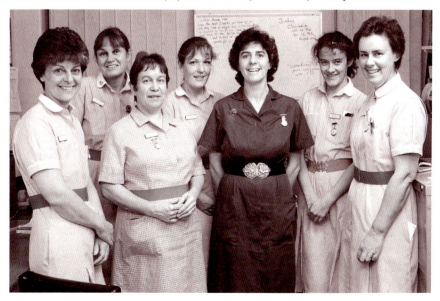

improvements funded from savings achieved following the introduction of a system have been found a good way to secure co-operation. These are highly visible yet relatively inexpensive.

115. The timing and pace of systems implementation should be decided in consultation with the wards. It is unlikely to be successful if rushed. Once the system is in place, senior nurses and managers should go out of their way to show that they are aware of how it is being used and what it is showing. But they need to do this in a way that does not destroy feelings of 'ownership'. They should actively encourage research by ward staff using information from the system and, where appropriate, facilitate the implementation of its findings. Small changes should be made at an early stage rather than waiting until evidence has been collected over a protracted period. Staff commitment and enthusiasm must be sustained beyond the initial implementation phase by engendering a continually renewed sense of system ownership.

(ii) ADEQUATE EDUCATION

116. Adequate resources must be devoted to educating nurses to use information and supporting their use of nursing management systems (Box G). It may be necessary temporarily to provide wards with additional staff to enable nurses to participate in courses. It is necessary to ensure that nurses subsequently have adequate time to benefit from such education. Education should be designed to develop nurses' appreciation of the potential of the system and how to use it effectively, rather than just to train them in the use of the computer. The project team should try to ensure that the value of systems continues to be appreciated once the novelty wears off, both by the nurses at ward level who are required to collect and enter data and by their immediate managers. This may require them actively to seek out and promote novel uses for the information provided. It is equally essential that all users appreciate that the system is an aid to provision of better nursing care but is not infallible. They must therefore understand what the system can not do. Also, until it becomes an integral part of pre-registration nurse education, there may also be a need for more basic training in computer literacy and keyboard skills.

EDUCATING AND SUPPORTING NURSES IN THEIR USE OF A NMS

— Provide each member of staff with an information pack setting out why a nursing management and information system is being introduced, how the system was selected and how it is intended that the information will be used, with a statement of underlying principles and a list of pitfalls to avoid. Include any articles about the way it is used in other hospitals and information on the arrangements made for further support and training. Ensure that new members of staff continue to get this information.

— Arrange for at least one nurse from each ward to be educated and trained as an expert who can then be used as a resource, a liaison point, and if necessary an arbitrator, by the other staff.

— Consider what training it would be appropriate to provide for ward support staff so that nurses time is not wasted on routine data entry or sorting out computer problems. In some cases, the ward clerk or another unqualified member of staff may have the aptitude to take on the role of first line technical back-up in use of the system including, eventually, basic retrieval and manipulation of care plan, workload or roster data required by nurses for nursing audit purposes.

— Arrange education and training sessions for every member of the day and night staff. Agree the minimum number of sessions that each must attend. Provide this training away from the ward. Agree how nursing cover will be maintained. Ensure that training in basic computer literacy and keyboard skills is also made available to those who require it. Make adequate provision for training staff recruited or transferred to the ward after the system has been implemented.

— Keep an education and training register so that gaps and further training needs can be pin-pointed and so that the amount of nursing time needed to implement and maintain systems can be monitored.

— Arrange for classification of patient care needs and the associated workload to be supervised by an 'expert' from outside the ward for the first fortnight. Establish a system which permits subsequent regular and random checks on reliability and validity. Involve nurses in peer and self audit in order improve the consistency with which patient care needs are assessed.

A Case Study:-

At one hospital studied, additional staffing resources were made available to permit training to take place away from the ward. Three project nurses were employed to support implementation. During the initial period after each ward was connected to the system, 24 hour per day support and advice was available. Following evaluation of the success of the initial training, a series of follow-up seminars was organised to help nurses and nurse managers gain a wider appreciation of the potential of the system and how it could be used to improve the quality and consistency of patient care.

(iii) APPROPRIATE COSTING OF PATIENT CARE

117. Research into ways in which patients can be most appropriately grouped prior to admission according to their predicted nursing care needs is currently in progress. It will not at present be worthwhile to try to be too precise. With the spread of resource management, it is likely that a far wider range of staff will need to use nursing cost data. Guidelines should therefore be issued on situations in which it would be appropriate to use marginal costs and those where average costs are needed. Costs may need to be based on the care ideally needed by patients, or on the care planned for those patients in the light of the available resources and current standards, or on the care which is normally actually delivered. For instance, if calculating the cost savings achievable by closing a bed, it may only be appropriate to consider savings in *marginal* workload associated with the reduction in direct care compared to the standards normally actually achieved. New services should normally be costed to take into account any additional ward overheads and the level of care likely to be needed by the expected mix of patients.

(iv) EVALUATION

118. The project group should formulate an evaluation plan, agreeing measurable goals and quantified targets, timetables and review dates at the time that the Statement of Need is finalised. They will need to ensure that they have sufficient data on current procedures and quality of care to evaluate change. The plan may need to be amended if use of the system does not have the desired effect or if there are significant changes in service organisation or strategy.

119. A number of questions will need to be addressed:

▼ Are the data entered into the system sufficiently accurate and complete for the purposes to which information produced by the system is used?

▼ Is the system training and support provided by the project team and by the system supplier adequate? Do both nurses and managers or clinicians using information produced by the system have a proper appreciation of its potential and limitations?

▼   Has the system met the expectations of those using it or the information which it produces? Do they find it user friendly and suitable for their needs? Have they any suggestions for improvement?

▼   Is the system being operated efficiently and in accordance with established procedures and guide-lines? Has there been a full security review of the system and has this concluded that patient confidentiality is properly protected and that data are secured against corruption or erasure?

▼   What use is actually being made of information produced by the system and how does this differ from what was originally envisaged? Is it possible to quantify or list changes and decisions that have resulted wholly or partially from use of the system?

▼   How have these changes contributed to attainment of the hospital and nursing service's strategic objectives, to improved staff satisfaction and better patient care? Have there been any undesirable side-effects?

▼   Has use of the system resulted in quantifiable cost or time savings? In retrospect how do the costs actually incurred and benefits secured compare with those in any option appraisal undertaken before the system was ordered?

▼   What changes need to be made to the system or the way it is used in order to improve its value? How can these best be implemented?

▼   Once these changes are made, will the anticipated on-going benefits be sufficient in comparison to the full operating costs to justify continuation of the system?

IN CONCLUSION

120. Nurse Management Systems have considerable potential for providing the improved information that ward sisters increasingly need for devolved management of resources and developing the quality of care. But, in the rush to meet Resource Management timetables, systems are sometimes being installed without proper consideration of objectives. They may not reflect ways in which nursing in acute hospitals is changing. Once chosen, the scale of investment in these systems may mean that they inhibit further change which could improve the quality of care delivered to patients. Attention to the recommendations made in this report and by the Commission's local auditors should help to avoid some of the pitfalls. However much more needs to be done to evaluate the wider effects of existing systems and improve the ways in which they are used.

Summary of Recommendations:

FOR HOSPITALS THAT HAVE NOT YET FINALISED THEIR CHOICE OF NURSING SYSTEM:

INITIAL ASSESSMENT OF INFORMATION NEEDS

(a) Plan systems in the context of the overall development of the nursing service to meet the needs of patients (paragraphs 12, 13, 22, 23).

(b) Emphasise the provision of information for nurses, about patients, information which will help them plan work and review their practice, and information about resources to help them manage efficiently. Do not design information systems primarily to enable managers to check up on how nurses are doing their jobs or to move 'pairs of hands' around the hospital (paragraphs 14, 24, 25).

(c) Review current practice before system requirements are specified (paragraphs 15, 26).

(d) Set clear prioritised objectives for information systems reflecting their expected contribution to improved efficiency and quality of patient care Consider how additional information would be used before deciding what data are required or how they should be processed and presented (paragraphs 16, 17, 27, 28, 29).

(e) Choose a computerised system only if it is the most cost-effective way of meeting your objectives at present (paragraphs 18, 30, 31).

(f) Include in your considerations a realistic estimate of the cost of nursing time needed to collect additional data and operate the system during its lifetime (paragraph 19, 32).

(g) Ensure that plans are robust in relation to any possible changes in the provision and organisation of nursing in your hospital (paragraph 33).

(h) Check that systems and suppliers are currently able to meet your requirements including those for training and continuing support (paragraphs
21, 34, 35).

CARE PLANNING SYSTEMS

(i) Concentrate on how best to make care plans appropriate to the needs of
the individual patient and useful to the nurses caring for him, not just
on time savings and improved appearance. Ensure that options other
than full computerisation are considered (paragraphs 50, 51).

(j) Strike an appropriate balance between engendering 'ownership' and
minimisation of unnecessary time and effort. Use predefined libraries of
care but ask each ward progressively to review suggested care options
(paragraphs 41, 42, 52).

(k) Ensure that concise versions of the latest plan can be produced, but that
sufficient detail of care planned and actually delivered can be retained
on the computer to facilitate subsequent audit (paragraphs 43, 53, 54).

(l) Consider how patients can best be involved in drawing up computerised
plans.   Do not unduly constrain individualisation of care plans so as to
use them as a source of workload assessment data (paragraphs 46, 47,
55, 56).

WORKLOAD ASSESSMENT

(m) Ensure that workload assessment will be of use to ward staff, not just
managers. The emphasis should be on helping nurses to make better use
of their time (paragraphs 62, 63, 86, 87).

(n) Regard temporary movement of nurses to other wards as a last resort.
Agree at the outset the exceptional circumstances in which wards would
be asked to release staff or in which action would be taken to reduce
nurses' workload (paragraphs 64, 82, 84, 87).

(o) Strike an appropriate balance between consistency of workload estimates and choice of a system which encourages continued re-examin-
ation of workload patterns (paragraphs 71, 87).

(p) Before computerising workload assessment, check that the accuracy of prospective forecasts of workload will be sufficient for the use to which the information is intended and that other hospital systems do not require review before they can be used effectively (paragraphs 65, 83, 84, 85).

ROSTERING

(q) Computerisation can facilitate more flexible rostering. But ensure that rosters can be produced which are consistent with the way that the ward sister wishes to organise care (eg team or primary nursing). Do not sacrifice off-duties which enable continuity of care to be maintained for the sake of relatively minor time saving in compiling the roster (paragraphs 98, 104).

(r) Consider carefully for each ward whether automatic rostering has advantages over computer assisted rostering (paragraphs 94, 99, 105).

(s) Press suppliers to extend packages so as to enable a periodic analysis of rosters stored on the computer to be carried out which will identify the extent to which off-duties reflect patient needs and the scope for improvement (paragraph 101,106).

IMPLEMENTATION

(t) Choose a system configuration which minimises duplicated entry of data and permits access by the most appropriate users at times convenient to them (paragraphs 44, 49, 57, 80, 90).

(u) Do not rush system implementation. Its timing and pace should be decided in consultation with the wards (paragraphs 108, 115).

(v) Show that information from the system is used by managers and acted upon promptly. Do not postpone all decisions until a body of evidence has been collected (paragraphs 108, 114, 115).

(w) Ensure that resources and time for training and support are adequate. Educate nurses in how to use the system effectively rather than just instructing them in the use of the computer (paragraph 110, 116).

(x) When using roster and workload information to cost the care given to specific groups of patients, ensure that the choice of assumptions (care needed, planned or delivered, marginal or average workload) is appropriate for the purpose to which the information is to be put (paragraphs 111, 117).

(y) Ensure that systems are assessed against predefined criteria and to a pre-planned timetable (paragraphs 112, 118, 119).

FOR HOSPITALS WHICH ALREADY HAVE A NURSING MANAGEMENT SYSTEM

Some of the above recommendations may no longer appear to be of immediate relevance to hospitals who have already implemented a computerised nursing system. However they should be borne in mind when adding functions which are currently performed manually, integrating information from different parts of the system, or, eventually, replacing the system.

(a) Review the system in the light of changes to nursing strategy and practice, hospital organisation and management that have occurred since it was chosen. Consider too the implications of any changes in the relative costs of computing and ward staffing. Ensure that perceptions of how information is currently being used and by whom are accurate.

CARE PLANNING SYSTEMS

Paragraph 58 makes a number of recommendations. In particular:

(b) Ensure that there are procedures for assessing the patient centredness, completeness and appropriateness of care plans at regular intervals and for providing encouragement and support to nurses to improve the quality of care planning.

(c) Review the accuracy of information stored on the computer about care actually delivered to patients. Is it an adequate permanent record? Would it be of value to nursing audit?

(d) Consider periodically whether the libraries and units of care in use are consistent with latest research findings and are still appropriate to the settings in which they are used.

(e) Ensure that there are no unnecessary constraints to the individualisation of care plans. Ensure that any handwritten or free text annotations are not lost when plans are reprinted.

(f) Review periodically whether it has become feasible to reduce duplicated recording or entry of patient data.

WORKLOAD ASSESSMENT

(g) Ensure that nurses appreciate how to use workload assessment to make better use of their time and improve the quality and consistency of patient care.

(h) Regard temporary movement of nurses to other wards as a last resort. Agree, if this has not already been done, the exceptional circumstances in which wards would be asked to release staff or in which action would be taken to reduce nurses' workload.

(i) Check the accuracy of prospective forecasts of workload against retrospective assessments to ensure that it is sufficient for the use to which the information is intended. Consider whether other procedures, eg those for booking or cancelling bank nurses, need review in order to make best use of the workload predictions.

(j) Ensure that appropriate staff are used to enter data into the computer.

ROSTERING

(k) Ensure that the rosters produced are consistent with the way that the ward sister wishes to organise care (eg team or primary nursing).

(l) Press suppliers to extend packages so as to enable a periodic analysis of rosters stored on the computer to be carried out so as to identify the extent to which they reflect patient needs and the scope for improvements to the consistency and continuity of cover within existing resources .

5 Summary of Recommendations:

IMPLEMENTATION

(m) Show that information from the system is used by managers and acted upon promptly. Do not postpone all decisions until a body of evidence has been collected.

(n) Retain an adequate level of resources for continuing system support. Assess the need for wider training for nurses in computer literacy and education in how to use the system effectively to produce information which can be used to improve efficiency and patient care. Ensure that all users are aware of the limitations of the system as well as its strengths so that information is used sensitively.

(o) When using roster and workload information to cost the care given to specific groups of patients, ensure that the choice of assumptions (care needed, planned or delivered, marginal or average workload) is appropriate for the purpose to which the information is to be put.

(p) Ensure that there are plans for periodic comprehensive evaluation of the system (including all of the areas listed in paragraph 119).

References

1.   AUDIT COMMISSION (1991): *The Virtue of Patients – Making Best Use of Ward Nursing Resources.* HMSO

2.   AUDIT COMMISSION (1992): *Making time for patients.* HMSO

3.   GREENHALGH & Co / KINGS FUND (1990): *A step by step guide to the selection of a hospital nurse management system.*

4.   GREENHALGH & Co: *Nurse Management Systems – A guide to existing and potential products.* (Releases 1-8) (last revised Aug.1992).

5.   NHS Training Executive (1990): *Guide to the Implementation of Nursing Information Systems.*

6.   NHSME Resource Management Unit (1990): *Nursing Information Requirements – Identification and Computerisation.*

7.   KEEN J, MALBY R (1992): *Nursing Power and Practice in the United Kingdom National Health Service.* Jnl of Advanced Nursing 17:863-870

8.   JENKINS-CLARKE S (1992): *Measuring Nursing Workload: A cautionary tale*, Centre for Health Economics, University of York.

9.   REES S (1991): *How many nurses?* Senior Nurse 11:5, 31-35.

10. WHITNEY J A, KILLIEN M G (1987): *Establishing Predictive Validity of a Patient Classification System.* Nursing Management 18, 80-86.

11. BAGUST A (1990): *Dispel that old myth.* Health Service Journal 5 July 1990.

12. BAGUST A, PRESCOTT J, SMITH A (1989): *Teamwork Nursing System – Full Report of Comparability Study on General Medical and Surgical Wards.* NWRHA

13.   BALL J A, HURST K, BOOTH M R, FRANKLIN R (1989): '..*But who will make the beds?*'– Report of the Mersey Region Project on Assessment of Nurse Staffing and Support Worker Requirements for Acute General Hospitals. Mersey RHA, Nuffield Institute for Health Service Studies.

14.   BAGUST A, SLACK R, OAKLEY J: (1992): *Ward Nursing Quality and Grade Mix*.   North Western Regional Health Authority Nursing Department / York Health Economics Consortium.

15.   BINNIE A (1988): *Structural Changes*. Nursing Times, 83, No 39.

16.   BUCHAN J, BALL J A (1991): *Caring Costs - Nursing Costs and Benefits*. Institute of Manpower Studies.

17.   HANCOCK C (1992): *Nurses and Skill Mix*. Senior Nurse, 12, No 5.

18.   STONHAM G (1991): *Unfamiliar Language*. Nursing Times, 87, No 29.

19.   PEEL, V (1991): *Money is the root of all systems*. Health Service Journal. 31 October 1991.

Appendix 1

ACKNOWLEDGEMENTS

Thanks are due to nurses and managers in the hospitals studied and to colleagues in the United States (OIG), France (IGAS) and Sweden (SPRI) for arranging visits and supplying information.

Members of the Advisory Group for the Audit Commission Nursing Study were:

Jean Ball, Nuffield Institute for Health Studies

Heather Cawthorne, Department of Health Nursing Division[1]

Alison Kitson, Director RCN Standards of Care Project,
Director of Nursing Research, Radcliffe Infirmary

Helen Quinn, Nuffield Institute for Health Studies[2]
(formerly Regional Project Nurse, Northern RHA)

Prof.Jane Robinson, Nottingham University Medical School

Jane Salvage, Regional Director for Europe (Nursing), WHO
(formerly Director of Nursing Developments, Kings Fund)

Caroline Storey, formerly Regional Project Nurse, South Western RHA

Bert Telford, Director of Operations, Burton District Hospital Centre

Kevin Woods, Regional Planning Officer, Trent RHA
(formerly District General Manager, Chester DHA)

---

1   Sue Norman, Department of Health attended the first two meetings.

2   Helen Quinn also provided consultancy support to the Audit Commission's local nursing audits.

The project team was additionally advised by a group of ward sisters and nurse managers.

Comments on drafts of this handbook were also received from:

Adrian Bagust, Deputy Director, York Health Economics Consortium

Ann Brown, Project Nurse, Resource Management, Hereford County Hospital

Helen Derbyshire, Project Nurse, Basingstoke District Hospital

Jennifer Hunt, Chief Nurse, Royal Brompton Hospital

Maureen Little, Trent Regional Health Authority

Jim MacIntosh, JDM Management Services

Joan Mulholland, Department of Nursing, University of Ulster

Susan Pearson, Senior Sister, Royal Brompton Hospital

Richard Waite, District Audit Service

Wendy Wild, Project Nurse, Resource Management, Portsmouth Hospitals

and from the following organisations:

Department of Health

Institute of Health Service Management

The Patients' Association

Trades Union Congress

Welsh Office

The help of the many other individuals and organisations who contributed to the Audit Commission nursing study and who are listed in 'The Virtue of Patients' is gratefully acknowledged, as are subsequent discussions about areas of this report with nurses from North Western RHA nurses and with Greenhalgh & Co.

Correspondence about this report should be directed to Ian Jones. Other members of the Audit Commission Nursing Project Team were Jocelyn Cornwell, David

Shepherd, Sr Eileen Shepherd and Ken Sneath. Helen Quinn, who acted as consultant to the Audit Commission's local nursing audits provided on-going comment and advice.

Appendix 2

GLOSSARY

Acuity
The average dependency of patients on a ward. (But sometimes used synonymously with dependency or nursing workload).

Agency Nurse
A temporary nurse booked through a commercial agency supplying staff to hospitals, nursing homes etc.

ANSOS
An automatic rostering package with integral nursing personnel database.

Assessment
The process of gathering and evaluating information about the patient's health status, home and personal circumstances on admission to the ward in order that nursing problems can be identified and a holistic nursing care plan formulated.

Bank Nurse
A temporary nurse supplied to a ward from a list maintained by the hospital or unit of part-time staff willing to work specified hours on nominated days.

Care Plan
Prioritised plan of nursing care to be provided to an individual patient whilst in hospital, based on problems identified during the assessment and preferably drawn up in consultation with the patient or relations. Progress should be evaluated against goals on review dates specified in the plan.

Crescendo
An integrated nursing information and management system.

Criteria for Care
A widespread dependency based workload assessment methodology, including periodic activity analysis, usually linked to the MONITOR quality assessment package.

Cyclical Roster	An off duty roster which repeats after a standard period rather than being drawn up individually each fortnight or month.
Dependency	An assessment of a patient's ability to care for himself, eg with regard to feeding, personal hygiene and mobility. A broader definition is sometimes used embracing the patient's total need for nursing care including education, rehabilitation and psychological care.
Discharge Plan	A plan, based on an assessment of the patient's home circumstances and abilities, of action needed to prepare for satisfactory discharge and to put in place any services or aids that he needs if he is to care for himself at home.
DM-Nurse	An integrated nursing information and management system.
Early Shift	The first daytime shift, typically from around 07.30 to 15.30.
Evaluation	Appraisal, against a set of criteria, of the effectiveness of the nursing care delivered to a patient in achieving specified goals. The evaluation may show that his care plan needs to be changed or updated.
Excelcare	A computer assisted care planning and information system.
FIP Ward Nursing	A mixed dependency and task based workload assessment system with associated care plan generation packages (Ward Star/nCARE).
Funded Establishment	The number of staff at each grade funded in the budget for the ward or unit.
GRASP	A task based workload assessment methodology available in either manual or (as part of MISTRO) computerised form.
Handover	Procedure whereby nurses going off duty hand over responsibility for patient care to the new shift, telling them key facts about each patient; eg: impending treatment, changes in condition or care.

Health Care Assistant Support / Worker	Support staff, with locally determined pay and conditions, recruited on implementation of P2000 to replace the traditional learner service contribution.
Holistic Care	Care directed at meeting all of the patient's physical, emotional, social and spiritual needs as an integrated whole, rather than treating each problem or disease separately.
Individualised Patient Care (IPC)	Conceptual approach to provision of holistic care over the period of a patient's stay based on an assessment of each patient's individual care needs.
Late (shift)	The second daytime shift, typically from around 14.30 to 21.30.
Learner	Student or pupil nurse on traditional (apprenticeship style) course.
Model (of Nursing)	A conceptual framework for nursing practice, embodying knowledge, beliefs and values, adopted by a ward or unit as the basis of a common direction and ethos. The term is also sometimes used to describe the chosen form of organisation of care (eg Primary Nursing).
MONITOR	A quality assessment tool used to evaluate the ward environment and the process of care (including patient documentation).
NISCM	Nursing Information System for Change Management. A dependency based manual workload assessment methodology.
NMS	A computerised dependency based workload assessment system based on the McGratty methodology.
'Nurse Manager'	A nursing management system of modules designed around a rostering, time recording and nursing personnel package.

Nursing Audit	Systematic procedure for assessment and discussion of nursing care delivered to specific categories of patients on one or more wards with a view to evaluating effectiveness and ethical desirability of elements of that care.
Nursing Process	A systematic problem solving approach to patient centred nursing care, nominally adopted throughout the UK in the 1980s. The aim is to prevent, alleviate or minimise 'problems' presented by the individual patient. Components of the process are 'assessment', formulation of a 'care plan', its 'implementation' and 'evaluation' of the outcomes.
Off-duty	Nursing shift roster or schedule.
OnTake	Periods when a ward is the planned destination for emergency admissions.
Organisation of care	The method by which nurses and auxiliaries are allocated to patients or given care tasks on a day to day basis (eg Patient Allocation, Team Nursing)
Overlap	Period (early afternoon in particular) when more than one shift is on duty.
Patient Allocation	Method of organising care whereby each patient is allocated one or more nurses for the duration of a shift.
Patient Centred Care	Individualised, holistic care dictated by the needs and wishes of each patient rather than by the values or convenience of nurses.
PENFRO	A work study (task) based workload assessment system.
Pool	Central pool of nurses and auxiliaries within a hospital available for allocation to short-staffed wards (not recommended).
Primary Nursing	Nursing philosophy and organisation of care whereby the 'primary nurse', nominated for each patient on admission, as-

sumes 24 hour responsibility and authority for all aspects of that patient's nursing care during his stay.

Project 2000	Initiative to replace traditional 'apprenticeship' style pre-registration training for nurses and make consequent changes to ward staffing. An 18 month college based core programme is followed by a specialist 'branch'. Students receive grants instead of salaries and are supernumerary during ward experience placements, being replaced by HCAs.
Quality Assessment	Measurement of quality of the ward environment, nursing documentation and delivery of care, eg using a preformulated tool such as MONITOR.
Quality Assurance	Process of defining problems in care delivery, implementing measures to overcome them, measuring the results and reassessing the need for further action.
RADIUS	A computer assisted rostering system.
Rostering	Allocation of shift duties to ward staff.
SASHA	An integrated nursing management and information system.
SENS	A dependency based workload assessment system developed for South East Thames RHA. Can be linked to the HOSPEC rostering package.
Skill mix	The percentage of ward staff who are qualified. Or, more broadly, the mix of nursing skills possessed by ward staff, for example on a particular shift.
Standards	Statements of the levels of service or care related to specific topics which ward staff agree to provide. Normally accompanied by a description of the structure (staff, equipment etc) and process needed to attain specified observable (preferably quantified) outcomes.

Supernumerary	Nurses (eg P2000 students) who are not included in the funded establishment and who are not assumed to make a specific contribution to patient care.
Task Allocation	Method of organising care whereby each specific type of care is carried out by a separate nominated nurse.
TDS7000	A hospital information system including care planning, ward ordering and communication.
Team Nursing	Method of organising care based on allocation of each nurse to a team which cares for a group of patients for a number of shifts.
Teamwork	A 'systems' approach to workload assessment developed by North Western Region and incorporating a six point scale of quality of care based on nurses' professional judgement. There are associated strategic planning tools and information systems.
Telford	A frequently used consultative establishment setting methodology.
Time Out	Analysis of time spent by nursing staff away from the wards: sick, on leave, studying, or for example escorting patients or on other non ward duties.
Ward Clerk	Assistant, often part time, based on a ward primarily to obtain and file medical records, undertake routine clerical duties, answer the telephone and deal with straightforward enquiries.
Whole time equivalent	Total weekly contracted hours of full and part time staff expressed as a multiple of the standard working week (37.5 hours).

Note: This glossary does not attempt to include a comprehensive listing of all available nursing management and information systems or to describe all of the facilities that they offer.